MW00624213

FRIENDLY FIRE

A FRACTURED MEMOIR

PAUL ROUSSEAU

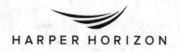

HARPER HORIZON

For my family

Friendly Fire

Copyright © 2024 by Paul Rousseau

All rights reserved. No portion of this book may be reproduced, stored in a retrieval system, or transmitted in any form or by any means—electronic, mechanical, photocopy, recording, scanning, or other—except for brief quotations in critical reviews or articles, without the proper written permission of the publisher.

Published by Harper Horizon, an imprint of HarperCollins Focus LLC.

Any internet addresses, phone numbers, or company or product information printed in this book are offered as a resource and are not intended in any way to be or to imply an endorsement by Harper Horizon, nor does Harper Horizon vouch for the existence, content, or services of these sites, phone numbers, companies, or products beyond the life of this book.

ISBN 978-1-4002-4796-7 (eBook)
ISBN 978-1-4002-4795-0 (HC)

Library of Congress Cataloging-in-Publication Data

Library of Congress Cataloging-in-Publication application has been submitted.

Printed in the United States of America
24 25 26 27 28 LBC 5 4 3 2 1

CONTENTS

AUTHOR'S NOTE

All names and locations have been either changed or redacted. The following does not infringe upon any nondisclosure agreement and is proven factual by both law enforcement and Public Safety reports.

PART I

HOLES

It is April 7, 2017, around 6:30 p.m. My roommate Mark and I are in the on-campus apartment we've cohabited for three years. We are best friends. I love him. No one else is home. We are on the couch, side by side, laptops on laps. Television on for white noise.

"Want to grab a beer?" he asks.

I'm not feeling well. Woke up with a head cold. A little throat thing. I absolutely do not want to go to the doctor. Camaraderie and a deep-fried pickle might just get me out the door.

"Groveland after 10:00 has got really cheap drinks for happy hour," I say.

"That could be fun. Wings sound good too. I'm trying to decide if getting a little buzzed would be considered a warm-up, or actually hurt my performance tomorrow," he says.

Tomorrow he is supposed to drink an entire box of wine and then participate in a bike race relay, dubbed infamously the Tour de Franzia. An event I would be a great spectator at, though this is with his other friend group.

"If it's beer tonight I don't think it would impair your efforts," I say. Mark is no stranger to alcohol. I have every confidence he'll do just fine.

"I kinda want to get buzzed up a lot today though," he says. As if baiting me for resistance. Who am I to tell him otherwise?

"I don't see why not," I say.

He turns the TV off and exits behind me, passing our roommate's empty room. Keith is at co-ed intramural volleyball practice with his girlfriend, Rachel.

I stay in the main living area, centerpiece of our apartment and great divider of each of our personal spaces. I'm writing a research paper for my capstone English class on humor and levity in speculative fiction. I realize I left a book on my dresser. I get up, take a few steps toward my room, and pause. I turn one hundred and eighty degrees, face the couch, then notice just how much of Mark's shit is everywhere. Bags, jackets, dirty dishes. Empty Mellow Yellow bottles turned chewing-tobacco spittoons. I'm not the tidiest person in the world, but the place is really turning into a sty. I figure I should do my part to clean up a little, set an example. It couldn't hurt. I lean over to grab something off the floor. A scrap of paper maybe, a dead battery, or guitar pick, I don't know. I don't hear it. I don't see it. But something comes at me through the wall.

INJURY

I've trudged through this story some thirty times now, to nurses, doctors, therapists, cops, lawyers, strangers, and one private investigator. I know the words. The words are simple: I got shot in the head by my best friend at school. No words over two syllables. It kind of sounds like a jingle, or nursery rhyme. But making the words come out is no fun. When I know they are coming, when I can feel it, I prolong the words as much as possible with lots of ums and ahs and back-of-head scratching. Once I finally get on with it, my voice finds a new register, as if my real voice wants nothing to do with what happened. I can't help but rock back and forth, elbows on knees, tense, shoulders high. I tend to get the shakes, kinking my neck weird. Talking is too quick, too sensory, too much all at once.

Writing is like a buffer against the physical aversion. It's control in a situation where I had none. I'm the dominant voice over everything that hurt me. It's a slick recovery tactic where I'm allowed to process things at my own pace. I get to muck about in the sandbox of the past and dig wherever and whenever I please. Most importantly, this chronicle affords my experience due respect and proper distance. A literal and figurative book on a shelf to be revisited in earnest, if and when necessary, but otherwise, on those good days, tucked away in my mind's library.

My post-injury brain wants to fixate and obsess. I can't focus for long, sometimes just fifteen-minute spurts here and there. The brevity of this book is an exact reflection, these fractured chapters a direct result. If I try to write for longer than my brain allows, it becomes hollow. I lose the ability to connect dots, maintain interest. I have to ask myself, what am I really saying? I rush to get it over with, unable to find substance. If I write anyhow, passing that point, ignoring my brain, it's murder, straight through the meat grinder. I become a fixture to the nearest couch, system overload.

A traumatic brain injury (TBI) is just that, an injury that traumatizes the brain, usually resulting from a violent blow to the head. More than five million Americans are currently living with a brain injury.[1] According to the CDC, there were approximately 214,110 TBI-related hospitalizations in 2020 and 69,473 TBI-related deaths in 2021. In the United States, guns are the most common cause of TBI-related deaths, above falls, motor vehicle crashes, and assaults.[2]

In many cases, the lasting effects of TBI—be them physical, cognitive, psychosocial—interfere with, if not entirely impede the ability to work.[3] In my case, I've experienced just about every symptom of a severe TBI. Problems with coordination and balance, changes in sensory perception. Difficulty thinking clearly, problems concentrating, understanding information, memory issues. Personality changes, trouble controlling behavior, nervousness, depression, anger, impulsivity. I qualify as Disabled. I identify as Disabled. In a world increasingly attuned to the damage of ableism, I want to add to this conversation and show what my disability can do. It is a challenge. I still want people to know what happened.

HOLES II

I'm blindsided, tackled into a pool of cough syrup. Soaked in thick liquid while wearing layers of yarn. My ears buzz, as if someone hit the monkey bars in my brain with a tree branch. The sensation becomes a chronic, caustic companion. I lift a forearm. My sight is a television color quality test. I stand and get a head rush. I'm fighting this sensory ambush and trying to figure out what it is at the same time. There is no pain yet.

I tell my legs to get up and walk but they've forgotten how, and I stumble. I am missing steps, evaluating the depth of the floor all wrong. There are no bodily boundaries. The material world is in revolt, continuously shifting around me. Is this the result of a natural disaster? Nuclear warfare? An earthquake in Minnesota? That must be how I ended up tossed into a couple of wooden dining room chairs. The fire alarm is wailing.

There is sweat or water all over my face. With two fingers I discover I'm bleeding heavily.

Mark comes rushing out of his room.

"Shit! Shit shit shit fuck. I didn't know it was loaded!" he says, one hand over his mouth, the other limply holding a pistol down at his side. I should be angry, or sad. But all I can think is, *I did my best. It must be time to go.*

He wants to help. He wants me to say something and keeps asking me to. But I can't talk right now. I am determined to go look in the bathroom mirror.

Mark disappears for a minute. I pull myself up. I don't know where the blood is coming from exactly. Somewhere on my head or face. I trip on silly putty feet and leave red handprints on the chair, the kitchen island, the walls. The path is random and disorderly, a child picking which house next on Halloween.

My face is strung with a thousand fishhooks towing five hundred bags of sand. My jaw is dangling like an undead decaying thing. I use my palms as kickstands on the edge of the bathroom sink. I hesitate to look at myself.

A hole in the middle of my forehead or through an eye would mean death is already happening. I'm shaky, weightless and top heavy at the same time, pinwheeling repeatedly in midair. I'm another dead kid.

I part my already clumping hair to each side. My bangs are a drawn curtain, below my widow's peak is a stage in a theater. I make way for the devastation by wiping excessive blood to an imaginary drum roll.

Nothing. Just skin.

I poke around the top of my skull, discovering an indent the length of a peppermint candy. I see only pink, red, and white. I move in close to my reflection and tilt my head like a holographic trading card to spot the bullet. Nothing glimmers or refracts. I look back toward the main room. Mark is carrying a red pouch. The drywall above our couch is pretty messed up.

HAIR

When they first got married, my oldest sister and her husband went to a psychic. Let's call this psychic Deb. No crystal ball or tapestries or heavy eye makeup, just a nice older lady from Burlington, Wisconsin, who loved buying lawn ornaments at renaissance festivals and smoking cigarettes.

They asked about kids and jobs and houses and happiness. They asked about my dad, who, according to Deb, wouldn't realize how much he wronged my mom and us kids until the very end. Then they asked about me, a sixth grader with only one thing on his mind: the guitar.

"He is desperate to know if he's going to be a rich and famous musician."

I imagine Deb took a long pause. Stared at the blank space between her and the newlyweds while she massaged her jaw, TMJ-laden from talking to complete strangers about their futures for God knows how many years.

My sister took notes.

Not a famous musician, though music will always be very important to him. Seeing a golden pineapple. Wealthy. Will help pay for my kid's college tuition. Hair. Hair also means a lot to him. He will be a writer who gets rich and writes about hair.

HOLES III

Mark leads me to my room and lays me down in bed with a pillow under my neck, ostensibly to minimize any swelling. He opens the pouch, a first-aid kit he purchased for solo hikes in California, and places pressure with some gauze.

"You must really fucking hate me right now," he says, speaking loudly over the fire alarm. There wasn't any smoke, I realized. The alarm was tripped, I think, because the wall it was mounted to had been shot through. Mark ignored it.

"No," I say.

"There is no way, dude. You must really fucking hate me right now," he says.

"No," I say.

He says he needs to get a better look at the wound. He says I should shower, so I tightrope over to the bathroom on my own volition, step by step, arms out to keep balance, because I trust him. He runs off somewhere again. I remove my clothes and start the water myself, sort of swaying on the balls of my feet, swirling like a glass of red wine, waiting for the shower to steam. I think about Mark's race tomorrow and wonder if he'll still feel up to going after all this. Hearing the front door open, I peek my head out of the bathroom and see him rush out of the apartment carrying multiple gym bags.

I find out later that, while I'm in the shower, Mark goes to the parking garage beneath our building to hide everything in case the police come. Into the trunk of his car, he throws the handgun he shot me with, three additional firearms, including a small-caliber rifle, a second handgun, and an AR-15, along with enough ammo to outfit a small militia. He hides the AR-15 inside a guitar case. Afterward, he returns to our apartment. I'm still rinsing off.

Blood and loose hair run down the drain like sediment. I have a haircut scheduled tomorrow. I consider excuses for the hole in my head, things I'll make up to tell the stylist: *Just cut around the gash.* I'm under the illusion that things can and will go back to normal. Perhaps even soon.

I dry off and carefully pull a clean sweater over my head, stretching the neck hole to get more than enough clearance around the wound. It's my favorite sweater, a minimalist black crewneck with my university's crest at the center, my clan. It reminds me of the fringe emo-skater fashion I was always a fan of in high school, but never wore myself. Oversized tops with extra slim pants that show off a name brand sneaker of choice. Since college, I put the jokey graphic tee to rest and really bought in to that aesthetic.

I lie back down in bed, head where I normally put my feet, and pain begins to loom. Liquid pressure; my brain is in a heat pipe. A headache to the bone, pain in my flesh like fresh cauterization by laser. The gut reaction is to touch the wound. I do. Parts of my skull move, and my eyes lace shut. It pangs as if the hole is one big cavity fixed with silver filling, and my fingers are wrapped in tin foil.

We get a knock at the door. I black out.

GHOSTWRITING

As a young person, instead of writing fiction and entering the mind of made-up characters—before I knew the term; before I knew it even had a term—I preferred ghostwriting. I liked getting into real people's skin, people I knew, and writing as if I were them instead, in the first person. I wrote short vignettes of friends and classmates. I kept track of our conversations, the setting, my sensations, the sensations I speculated they were having, and drafted out the scenes I found most stimulating. I wrote these in an ongoing computer document prophetically titled "The Messenger Always Gets Shot." Partly to sound evocative. Partly because, on some level, I felt conflicted about using others' stories to level up my own writing chops.

I rejected the idea of writing openly and honestly about myself. I felt uninteresting, like I had no problems worth exploring. I had self-esteem issues. So did everybody else. My parents were divorced. So were everybody else's. Somehow, Mom still managed to be my safety net and resource for everything. My ego told me to look elsewhere. I knew what I had and what others didn't.

I was accepted to a music school for guitar performance and recording. That had been the dream since I was eight years old: to become a studio musician, fairy-dusting layers of guitar onto famous people's generic music with a cigarette tucked behind the strings on the head-stock until I was discovered and could tour with my own band. Mom, the purveyor of reality with all the right intentions, recommended I go into dentistry.

We met in the middle with English, and off I went to a local liberal arts private university, courtesy of both federal and private student loans. A little over $100,000 worth of debt by the time I finished school. I could be an educator, copywriter, or proofreader, at least in her eyes. Something with a 401(k). Somewhere in the back of my mind, the idea of ghostwriting still had me by the throat. Writing celebrity memoir would be a thrilling life—just like the movies, and not too far off from being a famous musician. I could still dream.

In a course modestly titled Nonfiction, I wrote my first legitimate essay, something a professor would read and grade, bearing the name "The Messenger Always Gets Shot." It was a terrible montage of ultra-personal snapshots of my closest friends at the time, Mark among them. Some of the same themes have migrated here from the original essay, maybe even a scene or two, though hopefully improved since then. My first go at it was mostly a medley of poorly timed fart jokes and grotesque descriptions. Too much exposition. A little campy. I was a trailblazer, I thought. Surely I was the first person to write about this amalgamation of comedy and tragedy known as the Human Condition. Like a dweeb, I opened the piece with the dictionary definition of *cognitive dissonance*.

I'm embarrassed to read it to this day, but it does, in a way, work for me. The pages are weighty. The binaries feel magnetized. But it is a cheap weight. A dollar-store magnet. The title plays into the content by design. My subtle way of saying, yes, I know it is wrong to exploit tragedy for unearned feeling. It is a wink to the reader: Reader, I know—to write gruesome for gruesome's sake, and then turn to laugh, merits certain punishment. The essay was published by my university's on-campus literary magazine out of pity, I think. The students who ran the magazine were in my class.

HOLES IV

I only know these next details because of the police and Public Safety reports.

At 6:50 p.m., the fire alarm is wailing. The bullet tripped it when it tore through the drywall—same wall as the sensor. A tamper mechanism, I assume. The sound is contained to our room only. If anyone else in the entire seven-floor dorm building has heard the gunshot, they must have dismissed it as no big deal.

Mark lets the campus Public Safety officer in. I remain blacked out in my bedroom. Mark must have shut the door.

"Hey. Any idea why your alarm is going off?" she asks.

"I was smoking my e-cig," Mark lies. Help has come, but Mark is more concerned with his life fifteen years from now than he is with my life in the next fifteen minutes.

"I smell something burnt," she says.

"I had something in the oven for too long." Another lie.

"I'll have to write you up for smoking in the room," she says. No penalty for a first offense.

"Yep," he says. She makes note in her report that Mark is noticeably shaking. Abnormal, full-body spasms. His hands have it especially bad.

"Is there something wrong?" she asks. "Anything you want to tell me?"

"I get really nervous when I'm in trouble," Mark says. I believe he means it.

"Technically this is just a warning," she says, indicating her report. "But if it happens again, there will be more consequences."

The Public Safety officer sees Mark's empty holster on our loveseat, in plain view of the front door. Two steps inside, and she would have been standing exactly where I got shot.

"Where is the gun?" she asks. Mark's body probably goes faint, scratchy and gray like a freshly shaken Etch-A-Sketch.

"Car," he says. This is the first time he tells the truth since before the gun went off.

"Where is your car?" she asks.

"Off campus," he says. Back to the lies.

The officer takes a beat. Crosses her arms. Maybe rubs her chin or cheek, adjusts her hat.

"Okay," she says.

According to her account, she turns to walk out. But something new comes into view. A pool of blood on the linoleum. Above it, at least two stains on the wall shaped like claw marks. My bloody handprints.

"What's all that?" she asks, pointing at the ground. Her line of sight makes the hole above the couch difficult to see. But the red flags are everywhere. There's plenty of evidence. There's no need for a literal smoking gun.

"My roommate had a really bad bloody nose earlier."

You would think she might register concern, suspicion—*something* in her report to show that things were off. She has to investigate more. Right? There is no way this wellness check is routine, all things considered. But her report omits any indication that things are unusual.

"That should probably get cleaned up. Sooner rather than later," the officer says, exiting.

FRIENDSHIP

People are always so interested in how Mark and I met. They can't imagine a world where we weren't best friends. The answer is not all that unusual: it was the result of random room assignments from the university. Ours just so happened to be directly across the corridor from one another in Brady Hall, one of three freshmen dorms on campus. Although our motivations were wildly different, we both kept our doors open nearly all the time so that looking across the hall was like seeing a mirrored extension of our own surroundings. I didn't want to be labeled a loner, though the lack of privacy took some getting used to—but Mark, he didn't want to miss out on any of the chaos in the belly of what our RA, Ben, declared "the most fucked-up floor" he'd ever encountered.

Ben was quiet, even-keeled, kind of a normie. Well on his way to becoming whatever one becomes after graduating with a degree in applied statistics. Our floor had a high density of rich kids with influential parents, these students on a quest to push every limit before them—alcohol consumption, decibel levels, or any amount of nonsensical behavior that Public Safety would deem troublesome enough to jump in and defuse. Night after night, including weekends and holidays, fourth floor Brady was half ritzy Vegas nightclub, half prison-break maelstrom. Those party antics didn't vibe well with our RA, Ben. But Mark, on the other hand, was always looking to add his own brand of gasoline to any fire. He always seemed to find a way to escalate the chaos.

We would glance across the hall while facing our first college assignments, silently checking in, as though the creases by our mouths asked, *Is this as rigorous as you expected?* Our hands ran through our hair. *They want us to read how many pages by Friday?* The itch on our necks. *This paper has what kind of minimum word count?* Our communication was exclusively nonverbal, our friendship inevitable but still unspoken.

One day Mark was at his desk, shirtless as usual, puffing on an electronic cigarette and drinking bourbon from a fine crystal glass—as usual. I thought, *Hey, points for having personality.* He was reading on his computer, maybe something for Business Ethics or Introduction to the Catholic Tradition. I studied with the Lipton black tea I would pocket from the cafeteria. There on my desk was a ceramic mug with an accumulation of tea bags stewing in it, paper tags hanging limply off the side, making the whole thing look like a broken, upside-down hot air balloon. There I am, reading from the first fifty pages of *Dracula* or *The Tempest*, exchanging critical glances with the guy across the hall. I could tell he had had enough with the shyness. The coy anonymity.

He jumped from his plastic office chair and ran into my room, screaming wordlessly before belly flopping onto my futon like it would make a wicked splash. It did no such thing, and Mark flopped hard onto stiff, faux leather cushions.

Then a stillness. A silence. It was a bit odd. I still didn't really know him. So I took this as an opportunity to study Mark while he lay there dormant. He had that lean muscular definition of a featherweight UFC fighter; he was non-white, a few inches shorter than me, very handsome, with jet-black hair in a stylish mousse-assisted wave, wearing only silk-checkered boxers. He remained on my futon, pretending to be asleep, or dead, for a good thirty seconds, during which I considered poking the mole on his trapezius muscle but resisted.

At once, spry and jonesing with what I would discover to be a severe nicotine addiction, he bolted up and rushed out down the hall, screaming more and flailing his arms, looking like a flat-stomached hairless cat and leaving behind a full-body sweat outline on the fake leather. I admired his enthusiasm—if you could call it that—to meet new people. He was gutsy, adventurous, unafraid to have fun. He struck me as brave. I remember hoping, *Maybe that will rub off on me.* I'd like to think that, in a way, it did.

Mark came by again the next day, like a normal person this time, and added his phone number into my contact list under a false last name: a vulgar reference to female genitalia. (No joke—I legitimately thought that was his real name for a couple weeks, until someone corrected me after some ridicule, saying he'd played the same trick on them.)

"Let's get dinner?" he asked.

For the first two weeks or so of the semester, I ate my meals alone at bar-style seating in the cafeteria.

"I'd be down," I said, as I recalled great banquet scenes from movies of my childhood: The food fight in *Hook*, where all the food is colored in garish dayglo, wet turkey legs and neon green cakes; every Great Hall scene in the *Harry Potter* movies, the old-English warmth of a savory pie under magic floating candles. I knew how quickly a meal can familiarize people, make them like family. Just like that, first week of college. I'd be a part of a tapestry, stitched in right next to Mark.

Our table was an intimate open-mic night comedy spectacular between the two of us, expanding to three (Keith, who lived down the hall) and then four (Anna, a girl I met in an English class—we've been a couple now for ten years). But Mark and I were always the core of the group. We made each other laugh with dank memes culled and sowed from the day's Twitter harvest; Vines galore from when the six-second video app was in its prime; prank videos and photoshopped Shreks and smashed eggs and pure uncut internet. We found so much to bond over. Mark mentioned he was adopted, and that his adoptive parents were now divorced. I told him that my parents were divorced too.

Music was our love language. We made it tradition to wake Keith every morning for an entire year by storming into his room, playfully disrobing to "I'm Too Sexy." Mark once mistook "Funk 49" by James Gang for the *Footloose* theme song, and I berated him so harshly for that sin that, from then on, he'd mix them up on purpose just to watch me melt down. We turned anything and everything into a performance for each other. We would burst into song, a cappella style with kids' show choreography, no matter where we were, who we were with. I played guitar on stage plenty; I was used to having eyes on me as a means for entertainment, but never with such spontaneity. People never knew where to look. Didn't know if they could or should join in. *Is this normal for you all?*

I still found myself shy, hesitant, at times, but after a while, Mark exorcised all my inhibitions. Performance takes practice, and practice we did. He loved to be repetitive, purposely annoying, pushing buttons and getting in your face. A provocateur. I developed a long fuse because of him. Dealing on with his shenanigans, his nonstop scene-making, his impulsivity. But it all amounted to a self-confidence that I wouldn't have otherwise.

I wonder if he's still like this after everything that's happened, or if shooting his best friend in the head has dampened his boisterous spirit.

I was playing acoustic guitar the other day and remembered that Mark once had me video-call his parents a month before Christmas to show them my guitar so they could buy the exact same model for him. He liked the way it felt in his hands when I taught him the basics. He thought it sounded good enough while playing some open chords: G, D, A minor, C. He liked that. He had an ear for melody and picked up a baseline skill quicker than I thought possible. But he never learned how to bend the strings with nuance and feel.

I wonder if he still plays. I wonder if he thinks about me at all.

Sometime in 2015, we took our twin guitars to the beach, to Duluth, near his cabin. Keith brought his own acoustic too, though it wasn't the same as ours. We decided to busk, and opened our softshell cases on the pier, by the lighthouse. Two years later, Mark would use this same case to conceal his AR-15 after he shot me.

As he played, I threw a five-dollar bill into the open guitar case to make it look like someone had already donated.

We jammed for two and a half hours, cycling through the same five or six chord progressions. We took turns playing improvised solos, creating music that can scarcely be replicated. We gave, took, and shared with sincerity, our guitars having the conversations we could never.

Mark was still learning, but if I was confident enough I could teach him the tune in thirty seconds or less, we honored requests. On "Wish You Were Here," Mark used too much vibrato playing lead, eyes glued to the fretboard in between concentration and freedom. He didn't have complete control, but he was really trying. I gave him this encouraging look, proud as ever, when he did the bend lick I'd taught him that morning.

We made fifteen dollars by the end of it all and went to a smoke shop to buy cheap cigars. I still have a few of Mark's yellow guitar picks. The little cartoon turtle is starting to rub off.

HOLES V

I wake up alone in my room. From the other room I hear Keith and his girlfriend, Rachel. I try to listen through the closed door and deliriously connect the dots. From what I can gather, Mark has summoned Keith and is briefly explaining what happened: *I shot Paul—no, I'm not kidding. Come, now.* Rachel is arguing with Mark in the kitchen, ordering him to call the cops immediately.

There is something huge behind my ear, a bulge the size of a jawbreaker. It hurts to the touch, and I fear the worst: It's the bullet, that it ripped through my brain but slowed at the last moment, unable to break through the last bit of skull and skin. I feel around to confirm. There is no exit wound. I can't quit fussing with it.

I try to lean up slowly and eventually get up to walk. Everything is less wobbly but more painful now. First the doorframe—a checkpoint, something to lean on; and then the hallway, another checkpoint; and finally the kitchen, where the three of them are still arguing. I rest on a chair. It's from the same set as the one that broke my fall after the shot. Mark, Keith, and Rachel are around our island, eyes like flashlights. No one can believe I'm walking. I'm sure there's blood all over my face.

"I messed up. My life is over. I'm going to be scrubbing toilets for the rest of my life," Mark repeats again and again to himself, like a prayer.

We are all pale, though perhaps me most of all. Keith and Rachel, assuredly frozen in shock themselves, want Mark to be the one to call for help, to own what he's done. He insists he will, but does not. More time passes. Ten minutes. Fifteen. Tense silence. Rachel gives Mark an ultimatum: *Call now, or I will.*

Mark says, "Just hold on. Give me just a little bit."

Rachel starts crying, shouting in hysterics. "You shot Paul," she says. "You shot him. You shot him. Mark, you shot him. Call the fucking ambulance!"

But I know that my mom and I can't afford an ambulance to take me to the hospital. I'd rather hide my gash than make her pay a single penny. I was still convinced I'd be fine.

I press on the bulge behind my ear to see if it's still there. It's sensitive and swollen. I almost pass out again.

"I will, I will," Mark says. "Just wait. Give me another second. Just one more second."

I wait for it to kick in. Their voices are shallow, frozen ponds, little brittle things. Cracking into splinters and shards and smaller pieces. Sharp enough to puncture. Rachel goes to Keith's room to cry. I think it hits her even more when she notices the holes in the wall.

VARIABLES

For one minute, let's consider if I got my way and went to music school instead: "I'll play on the street, Mom. Or do YouTube guitar lessons." That classic headstrong stubbornness. Unwavering conviction with a tendency to rush. Overly optimistic to a fault. Alas, my band—Paul Wolf and the Full Moons—doesn't take off as planned. The songs are too atonal, unhummable. Never seem to build or go anywhere new. Paul Wolf is broke, in debt, maybe a little depressed. He may have to move back in with Mom. But he's doing the thing he loves. He was born to make music. For little or no acclaim, sure, but in this scenario the guys Paul Wolf jams with, the hippies Paul Wolf lives with, they in no way have guns. Guitar cases hold guitars, not assault rifles.

Or let's say the bullet misses me. By a few inches, maybe more. Maybe I'm safely in my bedroom. Close-Call Paul is like, *What the fuck was that?* He ambles his head around, his ears ring, he's unable to get a fix on the start or finish of whatever just happened. Mark runs out: *Fuck me, are you okay? Yeah, yeah, okay, but what the fuck?* Close-Call Paul doesn't get an answer, doesn't insist on one. When Mark lies to Public Safety, Close-Call Paul backs him up. *Yep, he was smoking, I burned dinner.* That Paul helps sneak the firearms out to Mark's car, carries the guitar case, naturally. No one will suspect a thing. Together, they patch up the holes with that quick-dry spackle, with loads of time left to laugh about this over happy hour at Groveland. Close-Call Paul has the luxury, the privilege, the luck of covering for his best friend. Hell, they're going to bond over this for the many years of their friendship yet to come. *That time with the gun—man, we were dumb fucks, weren't we?*

How about a universe where I was always getting shot. It was an unavoidable fate. But in this final imagined scenario, Mark finds it within himself to right the ship immediately. He is just as scared, but he wastes zero time. I'm in danger and he is loyal. And kind. And compassionate. Responsible. Instead of telling me to shower, he tells me everything is going to be okay. Instead of hiding his guns, he carries me tenderly to the couch. Instead of calling Keith, he calls the cops because he considers my life worth saving, and the valuation never once includes the threat to his potential future.

Power-of-Friendship Paul still texts Mark every once in a while: *Happy birthday you smelly saucy boy, hope you haven't sat in any gum recently, excited for the next* Elder Scrolls? They make casual noncommittal suggestions to meet up in person again sometime soon, but they never do.

HOLES VI

It's now just after 8:00 p.m. Keith, Mark, and I are still around the kitchen island with the intensity of a cult, the three of us forming a summoning circle. Not much has been said since Rachel left the room. Hands on faces. Fingers running through hair. Eyebrows hiked up as if stuck with tape. I am spellbound, in an unexpectant daze. Bracing my elbows over the counter to shift some weight off my slinky legs. Idle pain. Staticky stillness. Something is bound to happen soon. It has to.

I think: *Take everything in, friends, this is the last time we will ever all be in the same room together. We can't come back from this.* I know they are thinking it too.

Mark declares he and Keith will drive to Home Depot and get supplies to fix the walls. Wood filler and paint. Cover and heal the holes, make them blend in with hue.

"No one has to know," he says.

At the time, I think it's a good idea. Mark is as persuasive as ever. I don't really have a say in what happens next. I'm not even sure what *should* happen next. My mind is passively receptive to any and all recommendations. I'm unable to fully process what's just happened, but I'm through causing any more trouble. I don't want Mark to go to jail and clean toilets for the rest of his life. He is a smart guy, all things considered. He is the puppy you can't stay mad at after he bites your hand.

Keith says, "No way, are you nuts, dude?" His common sense comes in jabs like a counter boxer.

"Keith," Mark says, drawn out, a plea, as though to say, *Come on. I can't do it. You know this.*

"No!" Keith says, shaking his head side to side in wide, exaggerated swoops. "There is no way this is still going on. Call the fucking cops now or I will, Mark. You're wasting time!" Each syllable is another punch. Moves and countermoves.

Mark must sense the string holding the weight of this whole situation is close to snapping. Shaking, he reluctantly calls campus security, who call 911.

I prepare myself for whatever help may come by lying back down in bed, under the impression that I'll be easier to assess that way.

The cops arrive fairly quickly. Mark explains he has a valid, legal permit to carry. He asks what kind of trouble he may be in.

The lead officer is a huge man but he speaks softly, fielding the questions while tending to me and checking out the top of my head. Mark stands off to the side, asking if I'm okay every few seconds, apologizing in between to both me and the police. The officer tells him there won't necessarily be any criminal charges, so just take it easy. Another officer is taking pictures.

Mark doesn't calm down. He keeps taking tiny sips of water and for some reason asks permission to use our own bathroom, citing that he feels sick to his stomach.

No matter how many times I press on it, the huge bump behind my ear remains. I didn't know if they'd found a bullet or not. I worry it is just beneath my skin; I convince myself that I feel its shape protruding. I mention it briefly to the soft-spoken officer. It is not his number-one concern. My passive panic marches on.

A different cop does the math and figures out I was shot a little under two hours ago. He asks what the holdup was. Mark says plainly that he freaked out. Was worried about life with a criminal record, about expulsion, about ever finding a job. It's senior year; graduation is a mere month and a half away.

Someone says an ambulance is close. I say I don't want to go because my mom has no money. Mark assures me he'll pay for everything. I don't speak, allowing my silence to agree, reluctantly. Mark asks me if I'm okay and apologizes some more.

THE STUDENT AND
THE SUSPECT

After the shooting, just about every news outlet in the Twin Cities threw something together for quick clicks. Reading them felt dirty to me. Like a bad sex joke etched into the bathroom stall at a Kum and Go.

Most of the information was just plain wrong. Crucial context was laughably withheld. Other pieces altogether false. Imagine watching the NBA Finals, but every article the next day is littered with wild inconsistencies. Stats are skewed. Plays invented. The other team won when actually yours did. That's what it felt like when I read these articles. Guesses and approximations were thrown together and delivered with a staggering conviction of truth. As if two totally separate events existed in the same parcel of time and space.

Every article covered the basics: this University; that police department; here is a rough timeline of events. The students are both male, twenty-two years old, one from this city, the other from that city. Some included my name. None included Mark's name. The articles assured us that it was not an act of violence, which is debatable. They stressed it was an accident, which doesn't mean it wasn't violent. It was a very violent accident. The two are not mutually exclusive. We were assured there was no current threat. The weapon—never *weapons*, no one knows about how many weapons Mark had in our apartment—had been taken into police custody, as though the weapon itself were guilty.

We were assured that the twenty-two-year-old suspect (news sources don't typically name suspects before they are charged or arrested, and Mark was neither) was no longer on campus, which was untrue. We were told with confidence that no one was likely to bump into Mark by chance. Wrong again. Anna did just days later, overwhelmed and appalled, already overwhelmed and appalled from the incident, then doubly so after running into him. The police confirmed that Mark had a valid permit to carry when his gun accidentally went off in the dorms, injuring another student. Their concern was directed again and again to Mark's permit to carry. This, for them, was the salient detail. This, for them, made the whole situation a little less horrific, and somewhat okay.

Some articles emphasized that the bullet was fired through a wall. Or two walls, then into the common area. As though this excused anything. Some articles wanted us to know that the suspect at the time was not visible to the other student who was shot, that is, me. Most articles wanted us to know that the student—me again—was transported to the hospital. None of the articles devoted word count to the severity of the injury, the critical care and subsequent surgery, or, of course, the slurry of bizarre circumstances leading up to said emergency admittance.

According to these articles, all that was known for certain was that a gun went off and a bullet traveled through walls before making contact with *the student*. What word would best fit that scenario? The student was hit? Struck? Injured? All serviceable, though "shot" is probably the safest bet. None of these words were used. Instead, the word *grazed* was deployed, almost ubiquitously, in every article. The meaning of *grazed*, according to whatever dictionary Google privileges, is "to scrape the skin, or a part of the body, so as to break the surface but cause little or no bleeding."[1]

Ah, yes. Grazed. The bullet touched the gentleman's head lightly, shattering a portion of his skull bone before ricocheting onto the carpet.

A mere smattering of blood pooled and soaked into a pillowcase, along with some alarming red handprints on the wall. Besides, after reconstructive neurosurgery, the addition of a few metal plates and screws implanted in the head, it would be unscrupulous to call it anything more than an abrasion. Being a scuff, quite minor, an insignificant nick, the gentleman will struggle through a life of various physical and psychological residual symptoms—but never mind the severe brain trauma; we're in polite company.

Some articles mentioned that I was an English major.

HOLES VII

Among the quiet flurry of first responders in the apartment, my girl-friend, Anna, calls my cell. I answer and put it on speaker, hold the phone very, very far away from my head. She asks what the plan is tonight. Where are we hanging out? Doing anything? Going anywhere? I get giddy, almost. Not giddy with happiness, but excitement, sure. The way a microwave excites water particles to warm up a frozen burrito. For the first time, I'm about to break something catastrophic. My voice is vibrating with energy. I don't know how to say it. So I just do, the words creating their own kind of heat.

"Mark shot me in the head," I say.

"What?"

"Mark shot me in the head, from his room, through two walls."

"Do you need a ride to the hospital!?" Her voice is near breaking, a much higher pitch than normal. She is panicked and full of questions that will simply have to wait.

"I think an ambulance is coming soon," I say.

She starts to hyperventilate. I hear each incomplete breath of air, a swath of plastic wrap covering her windpipe.

"I'm on my way," she says, throat locked.

Anna is the one who contacts my family first. Per University protocol regarding discharged firearms and active shooters, an emergency alert is issued to all students and parents via text. In this case, the University informs all students and parents that the situation is contained and there is no additional threat. They communicate nothing specific to my family. No administrator or faculty member directly contacts my mom. She sees the alert like everyone else. On my phone, I will discover later her text: *Heard anything about this, sweetie?*

Anna gets my sister on the phone and tries to convince her it isn't a prank: "It's Paul. He's in trouble."

ZITS

Is this a good time to talk about zits?

For nine years, from twelve to twenty-one, no one saw my bare torso. No one but me and God ever saw the skin on my chest, shoulders, or back. My shirt was never off in public, I was never shirt-off, lounging around the house. I barely took it off when I was alone, even. Two fifteen-minute intervals each day was the only time my bare skin was ever showing—to shower, and routinely rid myself of my unsightliness with soaps and scrubs and caustic acids. Mom never saw it, even after she asked when I brought up seeing a dermatologist.

No pool parties, no hot-tub hangouts. No strip poker, truth or dare, or jumping on the trampoline with a sprinkler underneath. No sleepovers, no pickup basketball games. No sports at all. Not to mention dating. Because people would see them. The zits. I never pursued dating in earnest, knowing for certain I would be inquired to remove my shirt at some point. People would ask me out and I turned them down, hat in hand, with no explanation. The reason was hideous.

I am limited once again, post-shooting. No adult softball leagues, motorcycle rides. No crowds where things could get rowdy: floor seats at a concert, music festival mosh pits, dive bars after two in the morning. I am unwilling to risk a compound injury to my head.

It all began when I was twelve, just a few bumps on my shoulders and upper back. Where new hair follicles were blooming. It was something with my genetics, a missing letter, or one too many letters, which caused my skin to go awry and rebel. A simple glitch—it had to be—passed down from my dad's side. Though he never had acne himself, it ghosted through him to torment me. (I guess I also have genetics to thank for my abnormally beefy skull.)

In high school, this simple constellation turned into one of those pictures taken to show how full of stars space really is.

I hated the heat. I hated humidity, hot weather, the sun, sweating, and well-lit rooms, bug bites, rashes, cuts, any surface anomaly, of which I've had many. I got panic attacks—still do, on occasion. But now, post-shooting, it all goes much deeper. If I bonk my head on a low-hanging light fixture or graze it on a car door trying to slide inside, I lose my shit, wrapped up in how much irreversible damage I surely caused.

Because of zits, as a kid I became fascinated to the point of obsession with showers and showering. I would shower two, three, four, occasionally five times in one day. Still, now, in the shower, the pressure is off (no pun intended). In the shower, there is peace and calm, nakedness and freedom, even if only for fifteen minutes. I can do whatever I want while alone beneath the showerhead. I can think clearly and be myself. In the early days of recovery, any pain in my head would dissolve in that small escape of tile and glass.

During particularly bad waves of breakouts, I would go over to my sister's house to shower, under the impression that her city's water supply had radically different minerals that would be more beneficial for my skin. I would experiment: more or less chloride? I should have been my own science fair project: Profound Changes in Shower Water Have Little to No Effect on Cystic Lesions Considering Young Adult Male.

One day when I was eighteen, post-shower, after crying in the mirror, throwing my T-shirt limply to the ground, pounding my fists on the vanity, I asked Mom, embarrassed beyond belief, if she could make me a dermatologist appointment. And maybe drive me there too? Come with?

That's when she asked to see my skin. Thinking, there is no way it is that bad to make her son so flustered. It was.

"It's so strange," the dermatologist marveled when we arrived. "Your face is completely clear. At least your face is clear."

At least. At least I could hide it, if willing to give up so much. In place of quelling my stress, the constant sleight of hand only made it worse.

The dermatologist said I had a moderate-to-severe case. She gave me an antibiotic, two creams, and diet recommendations.

"You may not see results for a couple of months," she said. "It may get worse before it gets better."

I waddled to the car with my goodie bag of samples and prescriptions to be filled, full of new knowledge and hope.

My body turned into a topographical map of active ingredients. Apply a pea-sized dot of this cream across your entire back and chest. Shower with salicylic acid body wash, benzoyl peroxide acne treatment, let soak for ninety seconds. Repeat. Use a cleansing pad before bed to unblock pores, reduce pimple size, wipe away excess oil, remove acne scars, clear blackheads. Perfect—all this mess should be gone by morning. Remember, cut back on milk and cheese. These days it's fish oil and blue pea flower tea. Any home remedy or supplement claiming brain-boosting capabilities gets me hard. I take my health fairly seriously now.

I swallowed that antibiotic for a year and nothing changed. We switched pills to a different, stronger antibiotic. Swapped out one of the creams. Maybe try no dairy at all, they said. More antioxidants. Special vitamin soaps. Some with oatmeal, some with microplastics designed to exfoliate. Everything works in theory.

Then insurance stopped covering the prescriptions. Even though progress was slow, I had faith they could kick in at any time. Maybe even next week. That's what the dermatologist said. Mom could see the distress in my face, how heartbroken and destroyed my voice sounded. She paid out of pocket, sometimes three hundred to four hundred dollars per tube of gel or bottle of pills. Each would last about a month. The bills she paid from the shooting would make those prescriptions look like pocket change.

I hated myself, deeply. Hated my unclear, gross appearance. Hated the pain, the popping, scratching, healing, scars like little white breath mints embedded in my skin. Only for another one to sprout in the same place days later. A round, red weed. I hated the time it ate up, the time spent doing and not doing the things I wanted. I hated the excuses I made to shower, the lengths I went to rinse off. Then I'd look in the mirror and find no progress either way. I didn't look the way I wanted to feel, and it seemed there was little I could do about it. When I was sixteen, I made a pact to kill myself at twenty-seven if I was still unhappy in my body. Go out with the other misfit legends I idolized. I know that is stupid and terrible but an ideation that lives in me. More recently, I considered it again, from the stress of my personal injury case. The whole process felt like a slow, intravenous extraction that drew more than blood, vitality. It was a leacher of the soul.

Religion never played a substantial role in my upbringing, but it was always there in the background, so like a good Christian I assumed God was punishing me for growing up. I prayed, wagering with Him to let one simple bubble bath cure me. To bless this here water. I promised not to curse for a year. Not to touch down there, either. Anything. But nothing worked. I went on looking diseased, unclean, infected, disgusting, contagious. I didn't allow anyone to see me like that. I was putrid. Incomplete. Stuck in a gestation state, just like recovery. Not yet worthy of the beautiful world. Waiting for change, for years, is a staple of my life.

I brought this body, this acne, these dreams to college, thinking they were the greatest tragedy. Then I met Anna. She had written a young adult sci-fi novel about a female cyborg surviving in a zombie apocalypse. Anna had been to Europe. She liked PlayStation. She was beautiful and mischievous, foxlike in a cute way. She wore straight-across bangs, her malty brown hair the exact color of her eyes. Both shined slightly red in direct sunlight. She liked pepperoni-and-green-olive pizza and didn't believe me when I said her favorite was my favorite too. She wore clothes with decorative buttons and collars and interesting fabrics. She had a different sense of style. I had a different sense of style too. Her dad rebuilt a historic steam locomotive and now her family ran excursions with vintage train cars across the country. I needed to find out more. She was—and is—my priority. I asked her out. For once, for the first time in years, I decided that I would figure out my body later.

Anna never saw or touched my bare torso for two years, until I was twenty-one. Early on, she asked me to take my shirt off once, in her dorm. We were kissing. I had to say I couldn't. Not yet, I told her. She asked why. I didn't have a good answer. She saw me taking pills twice a day. I told her they were for an illness, I lied. For my liver. They were, to the contrary, hurting my liver. I could tell she was curious, but she never pried.

There was, in fact, a last resort that no one ever mentioned to me before. A medicine with side effects: the usual rash, itchy skin and eyes, diarrhea. It also caused major birth defects. As a result, I had to sign a form saying I wouldn't give pills to any pregnant people. But I got it.

It worked in days. *Days.* The root of all my anxiety was now gone—almost instantaneously—after so many years. I get an occasional breakout on my shoulders in the summer, some little white scars, and a large one on my head, but otherwise my skin is essentially clear now. I was free.

Acne was the start of my bodily shame and obsession with perfection, health. It was the start of my strange relationship with the medical field that would intensify after the shooting, and continues to this day: the guessing, the checking, the unreliable answers, the irrational cost, the perpetual question: Did this (the pill, the treatment, the ritual) actually do anything? Physically, I've survived. I'm surviving. But make no mistake: I carry secrets on my body.

HOLES VIII

Paramedics come in my room, and Keith, Rachel, and Mark recede from view. Medical personnel check my vitals, are amazed I'm talking, even brokenly. I'm talking because as far as I know I'm still alive, for now. An adrenaline mirage perhaps. It is verging on gibberish, but making noise is all the proof I need right now. I keep talking.

They strap me in a stretcher. I hate the attention. I am so embarrassed. Me, a handful of paramedics, and a couple of cops. We pass Anna on our way to the elevator. Anna. Anna's eyeliner is wet and runny. I wave goodbye, for now. For now? A cop tells her which hospital. She'll have nightmares about this moment.

We hit the first floor of the dorms and the elevator doors open, separating as if cranked erratically by hand. I would need many more fingers and toes if I wanted to count the number of times that elevator was closed for maintenance. We are lucky not to get stuck. My escort shoos away students and reporters.

Propped up on the gurney, I don't know where to look so I stare at my lap. Acknowledging it's there, unsure what to make of it. We rush by the front desk, the deer-in-the-headlights-faced residential hall staff, more students and reporters. I consider waving hello, but I never have before so what's the point in doing so now. Outside sits an ambulance parked in the horseshoe turnaround, and it's waiting for me.

BASKETBALL

In 2004, I still believed I could play in the NBA. Detroit born, my basketball fandom began with the Pistons—and at the perfect moment, at the height of their powers during my lifetime.

That year, the Detroit Pistons were in the Finals. We were getting new carpet in the living room. I was a kid on the driveway, in that beautiful uncontested thinking time that basketball provides where the body flows from move to move and the mind roams free. All synched up, totally as one, by the rhythm of a bouncing sphere. A sort of meditation, basketball has been a sacred act to me since I was very young.

I was working on my form, graduating away from using both hands to the proper crane's head flick of the wrist, pretending to be each member of the Pistons, one at a time, all at once. I was Chauncey Billups at the top of the key, point guard, with a pump fake, lobbing the ball to the low block. Grew seven inches, gained fifty pounds, I was Ben Wallace, center, grabbing the alley-oop and flushing it down on my six-foot rim. Okay, a layup. I was gassed.

A setting sun created a backlit suburban skyline, with a heavy spring coat of humid mist. Dead bugs in the flood lights, live bugs swarming.

Something is so satisfying about a basketball going through a basketball hoop, on any scale. The sound of a swish, so poofy and delicate, yet at the same time definitive, authoritative. The way the ball bloats the twine as it enters, the way the net curtseys as the ball splashes through. Basketball is sexy.

The game was about to start.

Dad had lugged our colossal, bulky box television to the adjoining Don't Touch Anything Room, what is typically referred to as a den, or *parlor*, if you're feeling saucy, where he usually read the newspaper on Sundays, and it was my job to refill his coffee cup on demand. My parents were not yet divorced.

Purple-faced, winded, bangs wet and matted onto my forehead in goofy triangles like a cartoon monster's upper jaw, I grabbed a Dr Pepper, ready to bunk down, feeling a surge of excitement in the pit of my stomach. Elated little bubbles were forming, building, and popping all around my small intestine. A feeling that came whenever I was a hider playing hide-and-seek, along with the urge to urinate. A feeling that came whenever I broke the rules. My own way, mildly. Reading with a flashlight in a blanket fort past bedtime. Taking a sip of dad's beer at the lake.

We got pizza delivered. Sat down together as a family in the *parlor*, our temporary hideaway from dysfunction. There, in the step-down living room just beyond our TV's new locale, a minor construction zone in sight, eyesore and potential safety hazard, with gym-mat-looking foam and some upturned staples, new carpet to be installed the next day. We were breaking the rules, breaking the norm. Squeezed together as a real family, for perhaps the only time in my parents' bleak twenty-six-year marriage. In the midst of dishevelment, we found harmony. That's basketball to me. Love. A pack mentality, and the confidence that it brings.

Billups finessed a fake behind-the-back pass, cupping the ball between his wrist and forearm. The defender took the bait hard, stopped, and reached out to intercept the air where he thought the ball would be, and Billups took the wide-open lane for an easy scoop bucket.

Mom *whooed* loudly.

"I've never seen that before," my dad said in reference to the flashy play.

Dumbfounded, I hunched over and got even closer to the TV, eager not to miss what would happen next.

On the other end of the court, Ben Wallace, the Pistons' defensive anchor, blocked a hook shot attempted by Shaquille O'Neal. Basketball at its best is this lyrical back-and-forth, an epic narrative. We decided right then and there to name our next cat Benny.

The PA announcer liked to overaccentuate the syllables stressed in De-troit Bas-ket-ball. Their mantra for victory. We echoed it back at the TV, arms up like at the cusp of a roller coaster climax, holding out the last beat until our breath ran out completely.

That year, the Pistons won the NBA Finals. I'm sure we had something to do with it.

HOLES IX

I am securely fastened in the emergency transport vehicle around 8:00
p.m., a paramedic on either side. One guy middle-aged with red hair, the
other younger with a small beard. Small Beard checks my vitals while
Redhead draws blood, inserts a drip intravenously. The sirens are on. I
don't like the sirens.

Redhead and Small Beard alternate asking me questions to see if I'm
brain-dead.

I speak in short staccato bursts from my throat, lots of time elapsing
for me to think between words. Like a jazz pianist allowing the background music to breathe and swell during a solo.

"What's your birthday?"

"December twenty-first."

"Full name?"

"Paul Jay Rousseau."

"Who's the current president?"

"Donald Trump, regretfully."

"Do you know how many shots were fired?"

"I think one."

They ask me where it hurts, if anywhere other than the obvious. I
briefly mention the bulge behind my left ear. Redhead nudges Small

Beard, then nods. Small Beard also nods, then looks out the window. I can clearly see Small Beard's nostrils flare in his reflection in the window. No one is optimistic.

"Can you walk me through what happened? Where were you when the bullet struck?" says Redhead.

"Living room," I say.

"Were you sitting or standing?"

"I can't remember. Standing?"

Something about that isn't right. Had I been sitting?

I hear Redhead whisper, "The bulge has gotta be the discharged round." He tries to explain the trajectory to Small Beard using his hands. The downward slope of the holes.

"Did anyone find the bullet?" Small Beard asks.

"No. I don't know," I say.

My most urgent, unprompted fear, confirmed. I just accept it. I'm a dead kid.

The emergency transport vehicle makes stops. I'm hoisted up and carried into the hospital, waiting, almost willing to die. I look at my lap again as I pass the urgent care staff. I don't want to leave them with the memory of my eyes. That would be very unfair to them, I think.

ANNA

Anna lived at her parents' place about an hour away, which meant when we would hang out, sleeping over at each other's house was the only option. At least, that had always been our excuse. Post-injury, she stayed with me at my mom's place as many weekends as possible. But her schedule was wonky. She'd show up at odd hours, leaving right when I'd finally realize she was there. I was often asleep, or simply out of it. She took the first retail gig that made her an offer, just to get some money in her pocket, fixing her attention on my well-being instead of her own. The events of April 7 delayed her successes after graduation too.

We were in bed, about a month after the shooting. A small table lamp was on. I wanted to sleep and Anna wanted to read. But we got into one of those talks, which meant we got into one of those moods, so neither of us got what we truly wanted.

She said, "I wish I would have been there."

And then she said, "I could have called 911 right away. Or maybe it wouldn't have happened at all."

She ran through the variables.

I shut my eyes. She was crying, I could hear it. Her voice was the background music to the scenes playing and replaying in my head.

I thought, *Enough.* I thought, *Why are we sad?* I thought, *I know how to fix this.*

With my pinky, I made a dimple on the part of her arm showing above the comforter. Then I glided up and booped her shoulder. Then I juked and made a move to boop the tip of her nose, maybe plug her nostrils, but she caught on, learned the pattern, and recoiled, now weightless. Nearly levitating.

She asked, "Why? What are you doing?"

I said, "The pinky is a funny finger."

She agreed and stuck her tongue out. I fake sneezed on it and zapped her ribcage. She roared like a baby dragon and swooped in to bite my nipple. I threw the comforter over her face and planked horizontally across her torso.

Our families both said we grew up way too fast. We lost some innocence, some faith in the world, after experiencing such a horrific event together. She could have left for every reason. Not wanting to play the role of caretaker, therapist, shit-wader for an indeterminate amount of time. But instead, Anna decided to stick with it. To stick with *me.* Because of that, we've become a rare contraption, one that is designed to land perfectly upright no matter how it falls.

We settled down in bed, awkwardly stacked legs under the covers like human Lincoln Logs, each grabbed a book, and read side by side fighting desperately to stay awake.

I thought, we would look so dumb if someone pulled the blanket off us right now. I knew Anna was thinking that too.

HOLES X

I am placed onto an examination table with thin paper lining. It is nearing 8:45 p.m. My clothes are sheared off by a horde of people wearing scrubs and masks. They work me over quick, checking for more holes. No one knows how many shots were fired. All they know is: this kid has been shot. They work, unceremoniously cutting my favorite sweater in half, right off my body to be eternally preserved in some evidence locker somewhere. Like ripping a Band-Aid off my deep, emotionally invested ties. I can't rep my school anymore. The universe just told me so.

A fraction of my boxers is left to cover me like a Chippendales loincloth. The rest is placed in an evidence bag labeled Flannel Undergarment. I am embarrassed by my pubic hair, the fact that I neglected to trim it now, of all times.

"Hospital. Yes. Yes. No. Just get here," a nurse says over the phone. She directs her attention toward me. "Mom is on the way."

"So she knows?" I ask.

What I mean is: *She knows I'm not dead, right?*

For some reason, the nurse misunderstands my inquiry. Mistakes it for guilt. Maybe it's the acceptance on my face, the weak timbre of my voice. Like I did something wrong. Like I am somehow responsible for my wound, as if I somehow caused the shooting.

"Oh, she knows," says the nurse. Face all puckered, each word a bigger and sharper stone being lobbed at my chest. What is she accusing me of, exactly? Does she think I'm in a gang? Does she think this the result of a botched suicide attempt?

I think: *You can't blame me for this. You can't blame me when you don't know the facts of the past two hours. I didn't pull the trigger.*

I try to string together a clarification, but concrete is filling my brain and halting my tongue. I want to say it was an accident. My best friend shot me by accident. I was just about to graduate from college. I love my life. Okay, maybe not *love,* but I was looking forward to change and hating certain things less. I was ready to be optimistic.

Before I can push out any air, the nurse leaves. Out a saloon-style double door with bubble port window. I never see her again. A new nurse enters almost simultaneously, much more informed.

"You're the first person I've talked to with a gunshot wound to the head," she says. "I'm going to ask you some questions, all right?"

I nod.

"What's your birthday?"

"The twenty-first of December."

"Full name?"

"Paul Jay Rousseau."

"Who's the current president?"

"Donald Trump, regretfully."

"Do you know how many shots were fired?"

"I think one."

"I'm going to check your vitals."

She takes a miniature flashlight that could double as a ballpoint pen and flashes it in each pupil. She says I have good blood pressure and I think, *This is the reward I get for eating healthy and never smoking cigarettes.*

I feel something pouring onto my forehead, like the cracked egg trick kids show off in grade school. Where a classmate would take a bunched fist and lightly tap it on top of another's skull, then slowly unfurl their fingers to give the sensation of a yoke oozing down their head. With two fingers I check to see what I already know. I'm still bleeding.

Different cops come in than from before, and I briefly think that I'm about to be arrested. Instead of putting me in cuffs, the officers take more pictures and ask if I'm positive the shooting was an accident. I say, "I think so."

"Any ill intent? Tension prior? Arguments?"

"No, no, I don't remember anything like that." I refuse to be the reason Mark gets in trouble. I refuse this, still unsure if I'm going to live to see tomorrow.

BASKETBALL II

A couple of weeks into my recovery, I was home, watching the 2017 NBA playoffs. One of my fun take-home prizes was debilitating sensory overload, so any television viewing required sunglasses to counter the blinding light, and foam earplugs pinched and loaded in the ears. Celebration—along with everything else—set to a minimum.

I'd left the Pistons behind long ago. For most of my life, and with more intensity than what anyone would deem healthy, I've been a die-hard Timberwolves fan. The Timberwolves are one of the losingest franchises in *all* of professional sports, not just basketball. And 2017 was no different, with thirty-one wins and fifty-one losses. But I didn't care who was playing. I was watching basketball. I was not dead, and I was watching basketball.

Mom sat to my right with the TV remote sinking in her couch imprint. Mom's new boyfriend, David, was in the loveseat to my left. LeBron James just drained a three-pointer after nonchalantly spinning the ball in the palm of his hand as if warming up pregame. I turned to my mom, smiling without teeth, eyebrows raised as if to say, *Would you get a load of that guy?*

"He is so cool," she said.

I nodded in agreement, then asked her an impossible, hilarious, ridiculous question.

"When do you think I'll be able to play again?"

I was hardly able to walk. Down at least twenty pounds over a couple weeks, and was instructed not to lift more than ten pounds or risk additional damage to my brain. My head hurt all the time. I could have a seizure at any moment, without warning—and there was always the risk that I could just simply fade away. I feared every headache would be my last.

"I don't know, honey. Probably six months, at least."

At this point, I went silent. The commercial break passed. Then David got up. We heard the rustle of him messing around in the hall closet. An *a-ha* traveled back our way and when he returned, he was holding the miniature hoop I had at school. The same one Mark, Keith, and I played PIG on before dinners. Our favorite nonsensical pastime for commercial breaks during *Star Wars* marathon weekends.

David threw me the appropriately scaled-down ball.

"Shoot it," he said.

I used actual jump shot mechanics and missed twice. He rebounded, underhand tossed it back to our make-believe half-court line. I threw again, changing form to fit the situation. I was adjusting. I had help. I was satisfied for one minute as the ball swished in.

HOLES XI

Someone grabs the back of my gurney and I'm carted off for a CT scan. I insist that I can hoist myself over to the machine without anyone carrying me. They say they wish every patient were like me—but not really, given the circumstance.

There's another new nurse. "I'm going to give you some iodine through your IV," he says. "Your face will feel flushed and you'll get the sensation to urinate, but I promise, you won't."

"Okay," I say.

He makes his way to a separate examination room and joins what looks to be a group of doctors. The instrument begins to hum in intervals, and a crescent-shaped part zips along above me. It executes a few passes over my head, and I get the flush sensation in my face and an unexpected surge of discomfort at the injection site. The first thing that comes to mind is whale watching, the *Jurassic Park* theme song. Perhaps a disassociation. A coping mechanism. Or perhaps it's because right at this moment, I subconsciously feel like a strange, scientific anomaly. A specimen to be observed. After a couple minutes the nurse comes back to find that I did in fact piss myself. He recruits some people to clean up the floor and leans over my supine body.

"We looked at your CT pictures. You are one lucky dude. Has anyone ever told you before that you were hardheaded?"

"Maybe." I ask if I'm going to die.

He says, "Probably not. Not from the injury sustained."

"So the bulge isn't the bullet?"

"No, the bulge isn't the bullet. The bulge is a very large hematoma, probably from falling after impact. Bullets bounce off you like Superman."

So: The bullet hit and fractured my skull, sending into my brain one large piece of bone and random shards, then bounced off. The very large hematoma was a consequence of hitting my head on a thick, well-manufactured, wooden dining room chair.

"Nothing foreign is lodged in your head," he says, "and based off the angle and location of the wound, the only explanation is that the round lost all momentum following the puncture."

So: after a duel with my head, the bullet rebounded onto the carpet, whereupon Mark then plucked it up and threw it in the garbage. The police find it and take a picture. I eventually see this picture. See the little devil. All crinkled and accordioned from the walls and my bone. I can't believe I'm alive.

The nurse asks if I want to check out the scans. I say perhaps later.

FRIENDSHIP II

Keith's entrance into my life wasn't nearly as dramatic as Mark's.

It was the first Friday night after Mark and I got acquainted. The two of us didn't care for crowds, and so were just hanging out in my room, drinking and jamming. I couldn't bring my guitar to the bar, so cheers to staying here.

Lulled by a Hendrix deep cut we were playing, "Power of Soul" recorded live at the Fillmore East, New York, on January 1, 1970, second set, Keith decided to pop in. Though I'd seen him around—all six foot seven of him—we made eye contact now for the first time.

"I'm Keith," he said, standing just outside the doorway.

His hair was combed back in a slick greaser fade. He wore gray skinny jeans, skateboarding sneakers, and a hip alternative black tee that barely made it to his waist since he was so tall, giving him the look of an employee at a Zumiez skate shop who'd recently hit a ridiculous growth spurt.

"Want a drink?" Mark asked.

"Sure." He stepped in with a "gee, you betcha" comedy hop.

We fixed him a Jack and Diet Dr Pepper, the same drink Mark and I had been nursing for hours.

"Dude you're really good at guitar," Keith said to me.

"Thanks, man." Some competitive bone in my body wants nothing more than to be the best guitar player wherever I go. "Do you play?"

He did. We agreed that Jimi's guitar tone on that particular track sounded just like hairy glass. This made us friends.

And our trio was formed. Our roles: me, the Bleeding Heart, introverted writer-in-training. Keith, the Wannabe Californian, just rolling with the punches. And Mark, the Cynical Jokester, center of attention. We became a Venn diagram of class, race, interests, and desires, each member overlapping in various shaded areas. Somehow, we clicked as a whole, with Mark as our guide. We decided right then and there to room together next year. Mark had enough credits and connections to get us into the nice on-campus apartments usually reserved for upperclassmen. We moved in and became a unit. Morning, noon, and night, an unholy trinity, them nude more often than not, hijinks all the time. Anything to be in that living room together.

HOLES XII

I'm wheeled back to the initial triage room. Minutes of silence go by until she comes in: Mom, eyeliner smudged, cold sore from stress already forming. Another life overwhelmingly changed in this instant, forever. I prop my hand up as an inadequate, matter-of-fact way to greet her. I'm a kid; she's coming to pick me up from a friend's house.

"Bullets bounce off me like Superman." I try to disarm some heartache.

"Oh my God," she says. She hugs me slowly, just around the torso to avoid any accidental bonking.

I can't really move so I just curl an arm around her back.

"Are you okay?" she asks.

"I don't know," I say. "I guess I'm hardheaded."

I squeeze my eyes shut but I am only just beginning to understand the irreversibility of what happened, the unknown of what's to come. The inside of my eyelids are bright-orange petri dishes laced with pulsating amoeba. Formless shapes replay the shooting. The sound I never heard, the fire alarm. I fall, then try to get up but falter. I'm bleeding, both in my memory, and the here and now, I'm bleeding. How on earth did it take me so long for me to get here?

The University sends a priest to pray over me. He is an old man, thin and fragile looking; he takes the whole "meek will inherit the earth" thing pretty seriously. His prayer sounds too much like last rites. Holy water and ritual gestures. Not in singsong, thank God. Mom covers her mouth. I stare at his clerical collar and the jiggly bit of skin hanging by it. He leaves while I overdo the *Thank You, Father*, really selling it with my eyebrows. Mom and I are both suspicious he is spying on behalf of the school.

My sister Alyssa—the middle child—shows up with her fiancé, Dan. I worked at his family owned upholstery shop for three years. Their wedding is just months away. Mark is invited, save-the-date card hanging up on his bedroom wall—though it was just recently shot through, so that's probably a no. Regrets?

My oldest sister, Krystin, arrives a little later. She's a nurse who works at a different hospital. Her husband, Lonny, is back at home watching their two young daughters, Alli and Aria.

Anna, not an immediate family member and therefore not able to see me, pretends to be my nonexistent third sister just to get in.

Everyone is crying gently. Most have their hands folded just below the waist. We make a familial U-shape around the CT picture on a wall-mounted monitor, my bed the centerpiece to the room, easy to crowd around. I work up the nerve to look at the screen. The top of my head looks like a cracked egg. My soon-to-be neurosurgeon identifies *that* white glob here and *those* little white speckles over there as internal bleeding.

I'm in need of a craniotomy. A titanium plate must be screwed into my skull to cover the hole. After that will be reforming the bone, roughly getting the pieces back to their original positions with scoops and rods and glorified tweezers. The neurosurgeon warns of the risks, mainly not waking up from the surgery at all—but it needs to happen. I listen and nod, fresh blood on my pillow already from where I'm still bleeding. Mom listens and nods and is the only one stable enough to ask questions. I am afraid but don't show it. This comes off as bravery, but it's not. The operation should take about three, three and a half hours. Surgery will be first thing tomorrow morning, given there is enough room in my skull for the brain to swell. The hole helps in this regard.

"I'll have you spend the night in intensive care to be monitored. Unless something changes, see you bright and early."

In the ICU, I get a tetanus shot in the ass cheek and we say our goodbyes, except Anna, who stays with the overnight nurse to watch me sweat and struggle for hours, unable to sleep. This is not my default most desirable sleeping position. I attempt to roll over, but inertia brings me back. There's no use. Dual IVs. Tubes and wires attached all over my hands, fingers, arms, and chest. I'm stuck in a medical web, and resort to staring at a particular patch of modular ceiling until my neck gets tired, then switch to a floor tile.

SLEEP

In the early stages of recovery after surgery, I was severely REM deprived. Sleep was impossible. When my body sensed that I was trying to relax, a bone headache would set in. Mechanical agony. Skull slowly accepting metal. I rolled and rolled and rolled, picking up wisps of comforter. I was that cardboard stick that cotton candy forms around.

Every foundational creak from the house infuriated me. Every click, thud, bang. Deafening against the non-sound of utter stillness. I considered the possibility that the noises were coming from inside my head, as plates of bone were finding places to set and fuse. To this day, the smell of memory foam makes me gag.

I would see flashes of whatever I happened to watch on TV that day, my mind trying to make sense of senseless things. The same two seconds of someone biting into a panini, or a basketball player running the fast break. Played forward and then rewound. Played again. The loops were maddening. I wanted to peel off my face, thinking the images would go too.

With the ambient amber lighting, it was never dark enough in the hospital to get anywhere near real sleep. I couldn't lie on my stomach or side due to the wires. At home, I had darkness and mobility, but still sleep evaded me. Those external hindrances were completely vanquished, and I had to face the facts.

I wasn't dreaming anymore.

Tylenol, that magic ingredient, helped. After that, simply time. These days, there are good nights and bad. The bad ones are when my heart thumps faster than the kick drum at a rave, uncalmable, a subconscious hypervigilance, an intense state of arousal. Bad when I wake up from a nightmare: someone trying to kill me in a deranged hybrid gas station murder dungeon. Bad when paranoia hits, thinking somebody is trying to break in, ready to kill me with a homemade knife/gun combo. But mostly good. Equipped with proper listening material, a Timberwolves deep dive or a comic hang podcast. Mostly good.

The first real dream I had after I got shot in the head was that I got shot in the head. I dreamed there was an active shooter on campus and that I had to get away. I didn't make it, woke up to my head snapping back into my pillow.

HOLES XIII

Sunrise, the day after the shooting. I'm changed and prepped for surgery. A pillar on my short list of fears. I can't stand gore, the thought of someone cutting me open. Twelve hours before, I didn't want to see a doctor for a sore throat.

I'm wheeled from ICU to a pre-operation CT scanner, and suddenly, there is my father along with me and the nurse guiding my wheelchair. Down the hall, down the elevator, down another hall. Walking and talking. I can't put a finger on the moment he arrived at the hospital. I don't know how he found me, how he knew what room I was in. I can't fathom his drive, crossing state lines so early for this, though I suppose he is used to getting up at four in the morning for work. From wherever he lives. Iowa or South Dakota. I'm not sure. I've never been to his place.

Dad simply blipped into my life again, as though by magic or teleportation. I'm unsure if this is my father or just a delusion. Stranger things have happened in the last twenty-four hours. It is bizarre seeing him in a specific, chaotic place, for such a specific, chaotic reason. Seeing him at all is such a rarity. I get oddly excited. Everyone will be here. Something is bound to happen. This is an *event*.

Dad sits next to me while I wait to be scanned and keeps talking. He talks like I'm a newborn baby, which is fitting. I'm certain I'll throw up some time today.

My surgeon goes through the rundown one more time with all of us present. I say genuine goodbyes this time, more genuine than in the first hours of all this, but not too genuine. I don't want to plant excessive worry. I carry a burden: if I'm shaky going in, everyone will be tormented the entire time and stuck with the thought that *he knew, he was so afraid, my God*. I'm whisked away fast. It's for the best. I wonder if that is a legitimate surgery tactic, to hurry before the patient really catches on.

Everyone takes turns touching my arm as I'm carted to the operation room. Dad jokes he will spare me the humiliation of a kiss.

The surgeon has a question: my hair. Shave off the whole deal or just around the incision? He feels bad about having to cut it at all. Says I have a really great head of hair. I know I do. I was born with a mop top and have only trimmed it since. I attribute a lot of my creativity to my hair in a weird, superstitious way. Deb, the psychic, clued into the energy of my hair, and Deb was no fraud. Plus, the only party trick I've ever found success with is my ability to look like any one of the Beatles at any given time.

I say buzz it all. I tell him I had a cut scheduled for today anyway, and that he is saving me a buck. On the upside, I'll look more professional when I get back on the horse looking for jobs after graduation. He laughs and says it should grow back by then. For a second, I think about what that means. The lengthy and strenuous voyage ahead.

I'm calm because what other choice do I have. I am completely sidelined. I got shot. That happened. Now *this* has to happen. This situation demands a degree of surrender. I'm reasonable, not courageous. If I had a choice, I would run away from all this.

I see the breathing tube to be situated down my throat. I imagine the tools, the procedure, the five-inch scar about to be made from just above my left ear to about the midway point on the top of my head. From here on out, everything will be measured based on *before* and *after*. I check for the hole one last time.

LETTER TO MARK

Dear Mark,

What the hell. That was weird, man. What the hell.

The part that makes no sense is that you're a smart guy. But in your room that night, you were what? Preening? Alone in your room? Proving something? A masculine thing? A power thing? A defiance thing? Look how cool I am, so big and strong, breaking the rules. Gotta wipe down my piece, tuck it into bed. You never needed any of that. You were funny and loved and charming, and you drew everybody in.

What did a gun make you feel that I didn't? A firearm. Our friendship. You made a choice. We were just farting around. I thought you were tired, dipping out to take a nap. In private, who were you? What was the allure? You could have been a fishing fanatic, fascinated with lures, casting for prey in the dry air of our apartment. But, no, it was a gun. One of many. You learned a lot from those concealed carry courses. I can hear the instructor now: "Not everyone can handle the responsibility . . ." and yet it's easier to obtain a gun than it is to change the address on your driver's license.

You've made no contact with me since the shooting. But we did see each other once since. Over a video call for some court thing. The judge didn't tell me you were going to be on screen; I started hyperventilating, looking around all crazy, sitting on my hands, rocking back and forth, making little movements that a trapped animal might make. All that, and you weren't even physically in the room. Afterward, my lawyer, pissed off on my behalf, told the judge that I needed a fair warning next time you'd be around. A trigger warning, if you will.

On the call, you were wearing a white dress shirt with baby blue stripes, buttoned all the way to the top. Something you probably wore at Easter mass once. The shirt was choking you. You always talked about having a wider-than-average neck and showed me the little extenders you'd have to use when going out to a fancy fundraising dinner for that nonprofit you organized, the one that covers basic needs and medical costs for the families of debilitatingly ill children. Your head was a water balloon pinched off, squeezed. Reddened and absolutely devastated. I've never seen you so sad. If someone were to poke you, you'd pop, leaving behind tear-soaked clothes in a pitiful and discarded pile on the chair. You never did cry on camera.

As my dreams slowly return, I see you all the time. The dreams are nearly identical, only the setting changes. We're at school, but it's either way into the future, all techy and whatnot with ginormous glass elevators, or way into the past in the attic of some old decrepit mansion. Whenever we get close this grainy diseased aura fills up the space around us, the air can sense the tension, the horror of what happened, though it's never explicitly mentioned. I don't think the universe wants us within spitting distance ever again. In these scenarios, we would quite possibly bring about the apocalypse.

I know you're sorry. We're past apologies. I forgave you the moment it happened. This shit messed me up, though, in some pretty diabolical ways. If every good memory I had of us was a lake, April 7 dumped into it a vat of toxic waste, tainting the whole body of water. Maybe a few things can be filtered out, but that lake is beyond redemption. Are you happy I didn't die?

Here is a thought experiment: It's five years after the shooting. Our memories of each other must be distorted, corrupted. We meet again, by chance, as we are now. Do we become friends? Truthfully, I give it fifty-fifty.

Paul

CRANIOTOMY

A tube is gently shoved down my throat. Someone holds my intravenous line like a beer bong. A brain-relaxing drug called Mannitol is administered.

With a mechanism involving clusters of labeled dots called neurotransmitters, secreting, jumping the synaptic gap, and attaching to tiny football goalposts called receptors in a very detailed and specific manner that I saw once on a PowerPoint slide in AP Psychology, I am encouraged to fall into a painless sleep. In this state, with my head placed in a three-pin Mayfield skull clamp, my head is shaved with an electric razor. In this state, I am encouraged not to mourn the loss of my hair. I offer little resistance, anyway. I am shaved, given preoperative antibiotics, and draped in the usual sterile fashion.

The Mayfield clamp attaches to the operating table to hold my head still during this delicate procedure.

The surgeon takes a ten blade, a very sharp and very small-looking hockey stick, to break the skin.

He makes a partial coronal incision, biased to the left, using the ten blade. He uses Raney clips for hemostasis, that is, to stop my brain from bleeding all over, and then opens my scalp in the left frontal region. The surgeon has assured me that he is after both a successful craniotomy and a good cosmetic result.

———

Later, every time I cough or sneeze there is this unsettling slosh in my head with intense pressure around my ears. Like someone tossed a sun-baked sno-cone against the back of my eyes and simultaneously plugged my ears with candles. Is something rolling around up there? I consider, briefly, mentioning it to a nurse, so I play it safe and ask Krystin, who is both a nurse and my sister. She will give it to me straight. She gestures the word *eek* with her mouth and says bring it up to the people here if it keeps happening.

Every two or three hours somebody new comes in. The hospital purveyor of faith and hope, the hospital troubadour, doctors, nurses, specialists who give me referrals to talk to other doctors. The most recent, Sarah, is an occupational therapist, here to test my basic brain functions, here to teach me how to live a valued and productive life post-injury. And she is definitely not in a good mood. Whatever the reason, Sarah is looking for someone to take it out on.

———

The skin and muscles are lifted off the broken bone and folded back. Next, one or two burr holes are made in the skull with a drill. Inserting a special saw through the burr holes, the surgeon cuts out the bone flap along an outline hardly different from those on a paper doll. The bone flap is lifted and removed to expose the protective covering of the brain, called dura. Skull fragments, compliments of the bullet, are stuck to my dura. Multiple comminuted—that is, pulverized—segments are removed. My brain flap is safely stored in a designated spot, like car keys when one arrives home from work. With the surgical scissors, the dura is cut to expose the brain—*my* brain. The surgeon looks at all those pygmy-sized pink vessels.

A supercomputer disguised as ground beef molded into a fist. When I wake up, he tells me kindly, "You have a very good-looking brain."

———

Sarah, the occupational therapist, introduces herself and I try to respond, but speaking has never been this embarrassing. I want to say, *Oh, I'm hanging in there, thank you, and yourself?* But free-flowing chitchat is a butchered slurry of consonants and vowels loosely strung together. It takes me almost a full minute to respond. Hearing myself stuck and confused, I'm mortified. I talk swiftly, tongue firmly planted in cheek, quick-witted and clever. Mom is on the couch pretending not to notice the change. I imagine we are both praying, *Please, don't let this be how things will be from now on.*

Sarah puts a tray on my lap, lays down a couple worksheets and some coins. Then we begin with general questions.

"What's your birthday?"

"December twenty-first."

"Full name?"

"Paul Jay Rousseau."

"Who's the current president?"

"Donald Trump, regretfully."

She doesn't grin like the others did.

"Where are you right now?"

"Hospital."

"Obviously. Do you know which one?"

I don't remember being told or seeing signs. I do not maintain an active database of all the hospitals in the Greater Twin Cities area. I've never needed to go to the hospital. I'm not reckless. I'm not sick. I don't play sports. I don't party. Also, I just had brain surgery.

"No," I say.

I feel bad for not knowing. I get defensive. I think Sarah is grading me and I'm losing points.

67

"Think," she snaps. "Make a guess." *This doofus, this dummy*, she must be thinking. I'm wasting her time.

We're in the Twin Cities. Fifty-fifty chance.

"Minneapolis?"

"No. Metro Hospital in St. Paul." Sarah is disgusted. "I'm going to test your short-term memory by giving you three words to remember. After the next few tests, I'll ask you to recall the words, okay?"

I sneeze while giving a shaky thumbs up. Brain sloshes against the inside of my forehead. I think of crash test dummies.

"Purple. Zebra. Clock," she says. "Repeat."

"Purple. Zebra. Clock."

———

The surgeon drills down. This drilling into the skull to where the bullet made contact is technically through an open wound. He excavates a left frontal hematoma using suction, irrigation, and micro instruments.

Since the brain is tightly enclosed inside the bony skull, neuro-surgeons use a variety of small tools that resemble larger landscape architecture tools. These instruments include long-handled scissors, dissectors and drills, lasers, ultrasonic aspirators, as well as computer-aided guidance systems. The surgeon picks debris out of my head like weeds in a garden.

———

Sarah picks up a pen and tells me to track it with my eyes. I don't know the desired outcome. Is it a pass-fail exercise? I'm extraordinarily dizzy. After thirty seconds she writes something down. Without any feedback, I try to regain my center of gravity by blinking a lot.

"Let's go through some money scenarios."

I do all right making a dollar out of two quarters, four nickels, a couple dimes, and ten pennies. I do less well with: if a baseball card costs sixty-seven cents, how much change would you give me? Anything that isn't a zero or five, I suck.

Sarah tells me to subtract seven from one hundred.

"Nighty-three."

"Seven from that?"

Frozen. Beet red. A kindergarten math problem. I'm overwhelmed. Embarrassed tenfold. Can I even count to ten? Mom is witnessing her son's brain damage. Watching an occupational therapist cross her arms at my silence. Roll her eyes. Isn't this her full-time job? Is she somehow devoid of empathy? She leans back in her chair as a form of protest.

"Eighty-four?" I say.

So, so sorry. We all know it's wrong.

"Seven from that?"

Mom lets out a burst of frustrated, hot air. She mouths to me: *I'm going to punch a bitch out!* She looks rabid. I wouldn't want anyone else in my corner. *You are aware he just had neurosurgery, right? Shot in the head? He is an English major for Christ's sake, he doesn't need to know numbers!*

———

The retractors holding the brain are removed; the dura is closed using sutures. The bone flap is placed back into its original God-given position and secured to the skull with titanium plates and screws. The joke is that I am slower now because I have additional mass folded into my head. I can't run as fast, Mom! We will laugh much later.

My incision incorporates the macerated entry site of the bullet. This area is carefully debrided using Penfield dissectors; that is, the dead tissue is removed and then reapproximated using suture and staples.

My incision scar will resemble the lightly massaged crease of dumpling dough. In some cases, the titanium may be felt under the skin. In some cases, a drain may be placed under the skin for a few days to evacuate blood or fluid from the surgical area. Muscles and skin are sutured back together. The surgeon sprinkles vancomycin powder over the wound and closes the incision in stepwise fashion using absorbable suture with skin staples. Many metal teeth bite down to help hold my head together like a bad animal with good intentions.

———

We move onto task management. Haven't I suffered enough? I am to designate an order of events for a simulated day. Sarah gives me multiple scenarios, some of high importance, some time-sensitive, some not. It's torturous. I am allowed scratch paper.

"You have a doctor appointment at three, birthday party at five, you have to cook and eat breakfast, fill up your gas tank, purchase a cake, pick up a prescription, and get fitted for new slacks. What order would be the most efficient and why?"

Honestly, I'd rather be shot again. (Not too soon!) I give it a whirl to appease her. She scoffs, taps her foot as I begin, truly trying to work it out and pick the right answers. My simulated day is royally fucked. I run out of gas. Eat breakfast at lunchtime. Show up to the party without a cake. Miss my doctor appointment. Ask for pills at the slacks store.

———

In a recovery room, I lie next to other people with similar clusters of labeled dots, by which I mean our neurotransmitters are attaching and detaching very specifically to tiny football goalposts called receptors. We are encouraged to wake up and feel pain again. Some people want to get back to it sooner than others. I wake up quickly. I'm asked to move my arms, fingers, legs, and toes. I don't remember if I'm successful. A nurse with a pen-flashlight asks me the usual: What's your birthday? Full name? Who's the current president? Do you know where you are right now?

I don't remember if I'm successful in answering.

I am administered medicine to temporarily prevent seizures.

The takeaway: I cannot lift more than five pounds. I cannot drink alcohol. Housework and yardwork are not permitted. There may be swelling, which would require a second craniotomy. There may be loss of mental functions. There may be weakness, or paralysis. There may be permanent brain damage, and associated disability. The results depend on the underlying condition being treated, really. It was a brisk two hours, all told. That will be $30,000 for saving your life.

—

Moment of truth.

"Can you recall those three words I had you memorize?"

"No."

But I can think of three new, not very nice ones. And that is a miracle among miracles.

LAZY

Before he made Mom and me leave our house, my dad told me: the greatest thing to invest in is yourself. He said that while tapping his pointer finger to his temple.

I had to sign the custody papers every child of divorce dreads. I was sixteen, crying at the kitchen table in the house I grew up in. I filled in the blank. And just like that, we kill off a whole half of ourselves. No more holidays with him around. No more breakfasts or ball. I will see my dad twice a year, once when he needs a good haircut and once more when he needs to get his taxes prepared. For the rest of our lives.

He then told me to take my hands out of my pockets, because people will think you're lazy.

HOLES XIV

I am wheeled to my recovery room.

Dad's girlfriend, Beth, says she likes the view from my window. She says seeing natural things, like outside, should speed up my recovery. Dad says yes, the view is nice, even though it's dreary out. He says I'm looking pretty good. The incision looks clean. His girlfriend agrees. My dad and his girlfriend are in the hospital room with me and his ex-family. It's a small room.

Dad often gets confused for Keanu Reeves when traveling abroad. Right now, he looks like Keanu Reeves if a scientist spliced some porcupine DNA into him, what with his hair styled the way it is. Messy and poker straight. It reminds me that mine is all gone. We do look alike.

He pulls a hospital chair over near my bedside. Holds my hand too tight. His space is in my space. Body too close to mine. Like something in his mind is saying, *This is how to show affection*. The whole situation is not unlike the time he walked in on me crying after he put down my cat without telling me first. Instead of saying sorry or offering any consolation, he complimented the song I was listening to, saying it was a fitting tribute to remember KC by. He always misses the point, by a mile.

Dad asks me to guess how many staples are on my head. I guess nine. He corrects me, nineteen.

"Same as my old jersey number when I played baseball," he says. Everything comes back to him. We are all narcissists.

My sister Alyssa called Dad yesterday, as soon as they all found out what had happened. Waited all the way to voicemail two or three times. Left a message on the last call to put it on his radar. He had been drinking, which for him isn't a worrisome habit, but it did hinder his drive until this morning. He eventually came.

It's time for me to eat, so Dad finds the hospital's cafeteria menu. I'm indecisive and not hungry whatsoever, so we order together. Something he'll want to eat. French toast and some sides. He takes the menu very seriously.

Dad gets a phone call. His ring tone, "Stairway to Heaven," blares. It gets all the way to the lyrics before my mom and sister and his girlfriend tell him to take it outside the room. A nurse gives him the stink eye in the doorway.

He comes back, grabs my hand too tight, and his phone rings again. Krystin tells him to shut the fucking thing off, what the fuck, it's too fucking loud for Paul. He nods but doesn't comply. He doesn't understand. He never came to my basketball games or my karate classes or my talent shows or Battle of the Bands. He didn't come to birthday parties. He didn't come to my high school graduation because he knew my mom's mom would be there. His phone rings a third time when the food comes. I take a small bite, but it's not happening. I'm not hungry.

Dad is around his kids again, all at once. It has been a while. I don't know his intentions today. I don't know if we all get along, or if we get along when we need to. He posts to Facebook a picture of my bandaged head, captioned *Seeing my children today*. He lives for likes. And this is a perfect moment to get attention from his small circle of friends from all walks of life, some corporate, some past relationships, some childhood friends. Mom makes him delete it. I don't think he knows what he's doing is wrong. Or he knows and is just a sociopath. But I love him; he's my father.

HOLES XV

My surgery just so happened to land on the same day we planned, weeks earlier, to celebrate Krystin's birthday. Party of ten. Someone had to call and cancel. In my post-op delirium, my mind takes me there anyway, plays what should be happening right now, had I not gotten shot a mere twenty-four hours ago.

We are supposed to be at the Yard House drinking a yardstick's equivalent of beer from tall, skinny glasses. Mom walking my nieces around the bar when they get restless. The salsa running out well before we make a dent in the chips. Half of us are ready when asked what we want to eat. The other half either say come back to me or point to a random menu item. We are toasting. We playfully demand Krystin opens presents before the food comes. We are sharing a sushi roll the size of a toddler. We are dashing salt on coasters. We are laughing too loud, talking boldly. Krystin acts surprised when the free dessert comes out. Either a piece of marble cake with strawberries, or ice cream with a molten fudge brownie. Either way, it comes with a single lit candle and a loose, botched chorus of "Happy Birthday." Our waitress teeters after a near slip, desperately trying to regain balance as if she were entrusted with delivering the Holy Grail. Faint candlelight illuminating her sweaty face. We all snag a spoon or forkful. Anna pulls out her card to pay; I say no, I got it. We all hug, announce the next time we think we'll see each other again. We go home intact if a little inebriated. We never once use the words *bullet, luck, accident, injury, surgery, therapy, gun.*

Instead, I'm throwing up dark green bile from the mix of antiseizure medication and opioids on a near empty stomach. My head is too heavy for my neck to support, like a baby's. Something smells different too. Like my pheromones have changed. There's this scent of latex gloves, hot breath, and freshly salted tortilla chips, oddly like those we should be eating right about now. The sides of my tongue taste metallic, reminding me of those first few days after getting braces in middle school, when food seemed to be factory blasted with copper shavings, silver dust, and iron flecks.

Our party of ten is here at the hospital. I'm much closer to unconscious than not. As languid as I feel, groggy and lethargic, time speeds up. Every few hours a nurse checks my vitals and it's like morning again. Like an entire day has passed by. For ages, I don't budge from this exact spot, on a bed with a call button. Marooned on Brain Injury Island: population one. Missing out on everything. I pray this is the floor of my quality of life. I'm afraid of what my new ceiling is.

My family orders pizza. Dad buys, I'm told later. They crowd around my bed with paper plates, quietly chewing while they watch me like I'm a scary movie or a modern art piece. My mouth is slack-jawed, only the whites of my eyes visible. I want to say hello, thanks for being here, but I can't push enough air, can't form my tongue, can't move my lips, can't remember how to connect those wires.

Mom leads the group out to claim that corner of the hospital wing with large, paneled windows and a nice view of downtown. She feels they are being rude. They look down at the park where I've enjoyed many a live outdoor blues concert. Is someone mentioning that? If not, what are they talking about? Are they talking at all?

It's raining today. It rains every day I'm here.

LETTER TO KEITH

Dear Keith,

You never reached out after what happened.

I'm sure for many valid reasons. Nervousness. The Midwestern tendency to not make a scene, to mind your business. Didn't know what to say, didn't know if I could handle it, thought you'd better let it be. Wanted to distance yourself from any legal ramifications. I think you were questioned a couple times. Once by police, once by the private investigator hired by my lawyer. Whatever. I totally get it.

But I wanted to let you know that I think about you a lot, especially when I play NBA 2K. We used to have those nightly face-offs, an ironclad rivalry: me and the 2000 Toronto Raptors with Vince Carter and Tracy McGrady versus you and the 2017 Milwaukee Bucks with budding superstar Giannis Antetokounmpo. Please know I often think about what secondhand trauma you and Rachael might carry from April 7, 2017; how awful it must have been to bear witness. It was an impossible position to be in but the two of you coaxed Mark to do the right thing, and I thank you for your persistence.

Technically speaking, we could still hang out. I could text you. We'd meet up somewhere for drinks. No alcohol for me, of course.

"How's your head?" you would ask, through an awkward half smile.

I'd unveil the deformity I live with, for just a minute.

"Mark sure is a wild and crazy guy, huh?"

"Have you spoken to him?"

You'd tell me Mark wished you a happy birthday last year and I'm both jealous and sad. Jealous because Mark legally can't wish me a happy birthday even if he wanted to and sad because I didn't wish you, Keith, a happy birthday last year; I was afraid to stir up old feelings and now you probably think I don't give a rat's ass about your livelihood, which is so not true. I care about you. But everything has changed.

"Remember when I tried to teach you how to dunk a basketball?"

"I was never tall enough," I'd admit.

"Remember when I played Cupid? 'Hey Anna, hear the song Paul is strumming? It's called "Anna." Interesting title, eh? Why don't you two grab some coffee tomorrow?'"

"You were the best wingman," I'd say. You helped me hide alcohol. You helped me clean vomit. These things were paramount then.

You would say, "Remember at dinner one time we tried to see how many bowls of cereal we could eat? I looked up from my Cinnamon Toast Crunch and said, 'I just diarrhea'd my pants'? And then you watched me waddle back to our apartment from the cafeteria window, waving and giggling?"

We were immature, foolish, a little perverted. We were boys.

"The funniest thing in the world," I'd say.

It had felt like we'd be doing this same stuff fifty years later.

But that didn't happen, not the same stuff, not anything together ever again. Maybe that's a good thing. Maybe now we can do more apart. We were so focused on ourselves. We were so funny, so clever, so self-centered. We weren't bad kids but we weren't good either. We supported various nonprofits. We occasionally donated clothing, food, and time. We didn't make a bad habit out of cutting class and we didn't do drugs. We separated our trash from our recyclables and disposed of them properly. But we were dark, insular, and at times unkind, mostly behind closed doors but sometimes in public. We put people down. We trolled. We wasted time. I'd like to think this was a rite of passage, a phase. But, hell, maybe we should have used our energy to do something better, cooler; start a sketch comedy troupe, make short films, write a screenplay. The world didn't need another trio of privileged and relatively intelligent boys fucking around for their own amusement, just waiting for something to happen. Well, something happened, that's for sure.

Then I'd touch your shoulder and say, "You can pick your friends and you can pick your nose, but you can't be friends with someone after they shoot you in the head." And we'd laugh and laugh and laugh.

The thing is, Keith, there is no us without Mark. And Mark shot me in the head. It's not a bygones situation, you know? Every second I saw you would remind me that I got shot, without fail. The two of us are only capable of the past, and I'm only in the mood for moving on. I hope you've moved on from this too.

There is a lightness to you that I'm certain you're unaware of, which makes it all the more miraculous. You made the funniest joke I've ever heard, to this day. Do you remember it?

Paul

HOLES XVI

I'm escorted to the bathroom, where I finally confront the mirror I've been avoiding every time I go to piss.

My ratios are all wrong. Sideburns overwhelm my shaved head. The surgeon preserved my facial hair. Of course he would. With one eye shut, I peek at my incision. It looks like a skin-tone caterpillar with silver stripes. It's hideous.

A shower is the goal today.

I'm afraid to slip the gown over my head. Afraid to wash the bloody fold of skin budding under thin bristles of hair. Afraid I'll get brain matter on my hands. Afraid my skull will fill up like an abandoned swimming pool during a thunderstorm.

Krystin helps me get situated. Each of the four chair legs has a little suction cup on the bottom. She waterproofs my IVs on each arm, making rectangles with clear medical tape that I believe is no different from cling wrap. Showering has been a personal and sacred act of mine for years. This is my first time with an audience. Just like when my clothes were sheared off by a hoard of trauma nurses a few days ago, pride and privacy are placed on the back burner in crisis times. My health has earned priority with the sentiment, *What choice do I have?* A mental shrug.

Krystin leaves and tags in Anna. Anna helps me undress. She announces she is about to run water over my head. My body coils, tensing up, goose bumps rising on my neck and arms. I brace myself. What will this feel like? Will it hurt?

Water ricochets off scabbed tissue. The drops make a low thud that only I can hear. It's different. Not pleasant. I tap Anna's hand as a signal to move on.

"You okay?" Anna asks.

I shrug. She hands me the detachable nozzle. I aim it at my upper back long after it has any hygienic benefit.

I use the handrail to stand, ready to dry off and get back in bed. I don't need to be reminded not to scrub my incision with a towel. The nurse reminds me anyway.

"Bet you finally feel human again? Nothing like a hot shower," Krystin says.

I'm not sure how much she knows about my past self-esteem issues, how much Mom has told her. But there is something universally remarkable about washing off past oils, dirt, stresses, and trauma. That cleansing almost feels like a rebirth. A regular baptismal font at the ready in trying times.

LINEAGE

My grandpa was shot in Iwo Jima, allegedly one of the first people to hold up the flag. He's not in the iconic photo, which in fact was a staged shot replicating the flag-raising, only this time with a much bigger American flag. When he was shot, the bullet went through one cheek and out the other beneath his ear lobe. He was a Marine. He survived, though he lost his hearing on that side by the exit hole, was awarded a Purple Heart and "another medal with a big bronze star and a smaller silver star in the middle," according to Mom. I never figured out what that one was.

My uncle was shot three times in the abdomen after picking up a hitchhiker. He'd known the hitchhiker, but not well. The hitchhiker told my uncle to hand over the keys and get out of the car. When my uncle refused, the hitchhiker pulled a gun and shot him. The hitchhiker dragged him into the back seat but left him to bleed for a couple hours before tossing him out near a hospital.

My grandpa died from heart disease in his sixties. My uncle died of his wounds at the hospital. Both were gone before I was born.

I didn't know those stories before I asked my mom if anyone in our family had ever been shot before. I'm not sure why she never told me. All I knew was my grandpa fought in World War II and my aunt remarried after her first husband died young.

They were more interesting than just their bullet holes, I'm sure. I'm more interesting than the bullet that hit me, I hope. I've developed a sort of kinship with my uncle and grandpa even though I never met them. This kinship is unfortunate but poignant, and not so rare. It multiplies exponentially as we speak. This is America's family tree.

HOLES XVII

It is morning—I think. Time has been acting fishy ever since I got shot. There is gauze wrapped around my face that gives me the appearance of a sickly, balding grandmother with black eyes. Maybe a grandmother that got bit by a radioactive raccoon. I look like that, sans any wacky superpowers.

I wake to the outline of Mom, my eyelids opening slowly as if by a crank-and-pulley system. With each blink, a new layer of detail reveals itself. Depth; shapes; a fuzzy, grayscale reality. The remainder of the room fills with color over time. And boy, is it full of color. And things.

Flowers, balloons, and gift baskets full of Easter chocolate and Fandango gift cards from people I've met maybe once, perhaps never, wishing me well. Such unsolicited kindness leaves me at a loss for words. I have heard nothing, received nothing, from Keith, Rachel, Mark, or Mark's parents.

"Hi, buddy," Mom says. "Your sisters went to the little shop downstairs and got you some things."

My throat is still too coarse from intubation to pass words clearly. I nod my head, careful not to be too extreme, envisioning my brain like that silver marble in the wooden maze I played with in grade school. Mom's holding a bunch of long, printed novelty socks. The way she's clutching them, her fist resembles Medusa's severed head, snakes and all. Mom holds up each pair individually like she's auctioning them off or modeling them for an infomercial.

"Superman," she says. "That's fitting for you, isn't it? Here's one that's argyle." She lays them down neatly on the end table next to my bed. "Paisley. And then we have stripes." She holds up a pair that's got little handlebar mustaches printed all over.

I lose it and turn my head to cry. I don't want her to see. The maneuver hurts more than expected. She grabs my hand and I wipe the tear away with my shoulder. A moment hits me. Those times I used to think about death as a kid, in the middle of the night. When she would always come by the third time I yelled *Mom*, scuttling me down the hallway toward her bedroom to sleep soundly until daybreak. I remember trying to match the rhythm of her breaths, unable with my childish lungs.

A nurse comes in and hands me mint green, nonslip socks from the hospital.

"For when you go home," she says.

Alyssa comes in after grabbing lunch and coffee. Everyone is in a better mood now that the surgery is done, and a success, to our knowledge. She notices the box first. A box, essentially unmarked, aside from an inscription made with black permanent marker reading, *To Paul*. Doesn't say anything, just takes a nail file to the packing tape. She has a hunch but is still surprised to see it in person. Alyssa was very aware how much I liked that hat. She knew the company, shared mutual friends with the founders.

There is this company that's all the rage now, founded by some kids a few grades higher than me at my high school—they make really nice knit hats. For each hat sold, they donate one to a child in the hospital, often hand-delivered by volunteers in costume as popular superheroes. A couple of months before the shooting, Anna and I went to a Timberwolves game; they were giving out limited-edition hats made in collaboration with this company to the first five thousand ticketholders through the door. Additionally, the Timberwolves organization made a healthy donation to a cause helping terminally ill kids. The hats were dope, a marvelous blue-green weave, branded with the vintage Wolves logo. We were too late. I was bummed, Anna was bummed, but they existed *somewhere*, and that was consolation. I talked about this hat a lot—too much maybe.

"It's real," I'd say, "somewhere out there, like Sasquatch."

While I was in surgery, Alyssa went on a mission to track down the hat. She messaged her friend, briefly explained what happened to me. They asked which hospital, and that was that. No further correspondence. Now today, this box arrives with an express shipping label to my room, containing not only the exact, pristine, limited-edition Timberwolves knit hat I've been foaming at the mouth over ever since I laid eyes on it, but six of them. One by one, the hats are claimed by my family members. I begin crying on instinct. Krystin encourages me to let it out.

"It's okay," she says. "Cry; you should."

I'm crying more about what the surgeon did to my head than the reason he had to do it. I only get one head. And now it is this ugly, demented thing. I'm ruined.

The time comes for me to walk around the hospital floor. The nurse has given me the greenlight, so long as the hat is clean, but I poof out the dome to keep the knit loops a safe distance away from the bridge of staples keeping my head together. I can't help but smile, holding on to my IV drip like a cane on wheels, attached by needle to the crook of each arm. Passing hospital staff who are happy to see me up and moving, every step feels like I'm pushing through dense gelatin bricks, but I feel vaguely warm and expressive. This is my team; these are my colors. It feels good to make a choice after so many poor choices had been made for me by others.

There is a window in my room, but I walk to the wing with the long horizontal panel of glass. Seeing natural things speeds up the recovery process, my surgeon says. I look at road signs and highway exits, trying to remember if I've ever passed this hospital on my way to anything else. Trying to pinpoint where exactly I was in relation to everything else.

PART II

HOME

Beneath the five-inch seam across my head is my prefrontal cortex, the epicenter that maintains planning and emotion. The tissue there is irreparably damaged. I no longer have control of what irks me or how I react to those irks. Small things become magnified. At any given moment, I fight the urge to cry, scream, laugh. I feel as though I've been grown in a lab in some alternative reality; as though I've been lobotomized by a railway spike; as though I'm entering the United States after a long time away, unsure what kind of citizen I am or what I should declare at customs. This is what it feels like to leave the hospital.

I move in with Mom and David, who just a week prior to the shooting had bought their first place together. I'm not supposed to be here. I should have graduated, should be on my own, poor, having to fend for myself in a shitty apartment. I should be healthy, capable, with roommates to complain both to and about. This house is beautiful. Open, and natural. Well-furnished to Mom's exact taste and specifications: tans accented by pops of gold and lavender, subtle changes in texture— seemingly more sunshine because of how she's arranged everything. It could easily grace a two-page spread in *Midwest Home* under the words *Bohemian Minimalist Royalty*. I'm spoiling it by my presence, and I'm ashamed. There's too much to do and I'm hopelessly sidelined. Eager but unable. Still very much struggling with speech and general ability. I worry David hates me now that I'm an indefinite add-on to Mom. I worry he thinks I'm entitled, that he regards me with malevolence. Mom assures me that David is just as happy as she is that I'm alive. Mom says my only job is to get well.

But we all know I'm a buzzkill.

I dance around words, pointing at things a lot. Perforated rectangle. There. Right there. By the kitchen faucet. Don't you see it? Please read my mind, this is awful. I'm stuttering again. Wipe. Big white napkin thing. I spilled water so I need this thing now, please. Mom comes to the rescue. Ah, yes. *Towel*, made from porous, absorbent paper. *Paper towel*.

Mom asks me if spaghetti is okay this evening. I click the start icon in my brain, trying to map my way to the meaning of the word.

Person, place, thing, or idea? Thing. Edible or inedible? Edible. I find it in a folder called Home-Cooked Meals and give a slow-rising thumbs up.

The master bedroom is on the first floor. I sleep there at night to remove the risk of walking up stairs. David sleeps in the second-floor guest room. Mom sleeps on the couch, spitting distance away from me. Mom says my only job is to rest.

My recovery is a never-ending sick day.

My recovery is the hour after dental work, but it lasts all the time.

My recovery exists in two states, pain and boredom; an excruciating bone headache or anxious boredom, unable to do anything I used to do for fun. Guitar is too loud. Basketball is out of the question. I play Nintendo Wii for the illusion of activity, make-believe exercise. Flubbing around on a pixelated nine-hole golf course, I enjoy the simulated out-doors, the pretend sunshine.

My recovery is making games out of monotonous staring. I had a popcorn ceiling in my first house, and whenever Mom would put me in timeout, I'd look for faces in it. There is a popcorn ceiling here, and I find a face that resembles me a little; I imagine Ceiling Paul getting into graduate school, or taking a year off to work, chipping away at student loans. I imagine he is not nearly as far behind as Real Paul, too stupid for work.

I take my pills with half an English muffin. Opioids, anticonvulsants. I take stool softeners so I literally do not kill myself trying to take a shit. I shower in the suction chair we bought from a garage sale. I make good use of cold washcloths over my eyes when it's not time for another painkiller yet. Simple things are forever different now, just by principle. Like brushing teeth. The mechanics are the same, the fundamentals. But now the teeth being brushed belong to a head that has been shot.

I feel like a slob, the worst qualities of a child and elderly person combined. I see the way David looks at the messes I make, notice his frustration as I drop everything. Spilled drinks. Broken glasses. Tousled blankets. I see the expectant look he gives my dirty dishes. Mom says my only job is to get better.

I hate that I'm unable to really work out, move right, help around the house.

I listen to *Nacho Libre* on Netflix with my eyes closed to ward off overstimulation and burst into tears by the end. It's a quirky, lighthearted movie, grounded in sincerity, about a cook played by Jack Black who works at a monastery/orphanage and leads a double life as a luchador. Professional wrestling is frowned upon within the community. Once his intentions change from fame and fortune to helping the orphans, he becomes successful, but most of all, genuinely happy. I see parallels. I discover that *Nacho Libre* scored a 40 percent on Rotten Tomatoes, yet it has moved me in ways I'd not thought possible, and *I've seen it before*.

Things are acting differently. *I'm* reacting differently. My defenses are down.

Mom is home as much as she can be. Her coworkers donated and pooled together their PTO. One coworker gave her a ring, a memento of her own son, who passed away earlier in the year unexpectedly, a gesture that makes Mom break down all over again. She cooks my meals. Does my laundry. Cleans my placemat. Gives me blankets. She watches me walk to the bathroom out of the corner of her eye, making sure I don't slip on the hardwood, which would naturally cause my head to crack. A tempered chocolate dome broken with a dessert spoon.

Someone always seems to be dropping in. My sisters trade days. I know that everyone's enthusiasm will wear off over time. I'm often out of commission, supine on a couch, either with a hood or pillow or blanket over my face. I look through the stitches and imagine what I would be doing at school, listening to my family's conversations like a child in the 1920s. Hearing everything but expected to be dutifully silent. At this point, it's as close to sleep as I can get.

I'm deathly afraid of zoning out—if left to its own devices, my brain, with instruction from the traumatic brain injury rulebook, could cause me to have a seizure. Or that I'll just fade out and die. I consciously stay in my own head, tentpole myself to the earth, and avoid drifting off like a piece of tissue paper over a roaring flame. I don't want to convulse. I don't want my eyes to roll back. I don't want to bite my tongue in lieu of choking on it. I don't want someone to reach back for my tongue while it is blocking my windpipe. I don't want to look scary. And I definitely don't want to be on the floor.

HOMEWORK

I wanted to go back to school. Immediately. I had been forcibly removed, unable to hit the end of college in stride. Robbed of graduation jitters, the communal *are we ready for this?* with friends and classmates. I didn't get to make those memories. And I'd be forever absent in theirs. I should have been applying for jobs and internships, but there was no way my mind or body could physically handle it. I remember thinking I'd wear a beanie to any future interviews so I wouldn't have to explain the mess on my head.

On social media, my friends and classmates were doing readings in the University library next to big, beautiful stained-glass windows and worn leather couches, winning annual workshop awards, having fun at school, listening to tunes in the quad, kicking a soccer ball around—together. The stuff that would become nostalgic years later. Meanwhile, I was swinging a Wii-mote sloppily at digital tennis balls, on the verge of tears, continuously losing against a computer doubles pair named Yoshi and Haru. Four years of hard work at a university for nothing. I felt erased by the school, left behind to rot.

My professors and classmates assumed I was cutting class. Where is Paul? This isn't like him. Mom and Anna took it upon themselves to correct the narrative: Yes, as I said, it was a lot more severe than first mentioned; yes, it required surgery. No, Paul didn't get grazed in the shoulder or clipped on the leg. Surgery. Yes, neurosurgery. Neuro, Greek for "Paul got shot in the head, he is recuperating, he can't write this email for himself, let alone a research paper." What do I have to do for you to understand that? They made mention of past performances, my studious history. Dean's list all four years. He has an A in your class as it stands, kind Sir or Madam. We would really appreciate any accommodations.

How this task fell to Mom and Anna, I haven't a clue. What began as an askance head tilt toward the response from the University had become full-body animosity.

I never wanted bad blood with the school. I simply wanted a little *help*.

I had major cognitive deficiencies. My mother was helping me relearn the order of the months. The months themselves. I also had a personal injury case, which made progress—or at least the show of progress—my enemy. Any improvement, any impression that I wasn't dumb and brain damaged, could undermine my case: Look! He's using that hunk of meat beneath his skull just fine! Like it never happened! Good as new! He doesn't need any money for medical bills or pain or suffering or any possible long-term effects we can't conceivably know the full extent of now! He knows his months!

At the same time, school was very important to me. I was forced to try to finish my degree in secret.

At first, I snuck onto the University's online homework portal and attempted some assignments in vain. With no lock on my bedroom door, I would angle the laptop in such a way where Mom would have to take a few steps to see the screen, granting me enough of a buffer to switch tabs to something else. I'm positive Mom would rather find me looking at porn than trying, and failing, to use my brain. In those early days, she told me I was pushing myself too hard. Relearning the alphabet by tearing through as many George Saunders stories as I could stuff in my cranium, reading his first collection *CivilWarLand In Bad Decline* a thousand times over. She'd watch me hold the bridge of my nose, squeeze my eyes shut. Then tell me to drop it, take a break, just give it time.

Reading was painful. I would scan the pages like a Pac-Man who ate printed letters instead of little yellow pellets, and he'd get full after about nine or ten. Eventually, though, my persistence wore Mom down. She didn't want to snuff out my hope entirely. Since I was technically no longer street legal, a neurologist advised to take arcade-style simulated driving courses before getting back behind the wheel, something I never did, Mom drove me to the one class of my choosing at school. A final shebang. A bit of closure. I chose a three-hour night class, my capstone creative writing workshop. Mom dropped me off and waited for me in a Panera down the road until it was over.

On campus, in the dark, with only a few souls scattered about, I pretended I wasn't at the school where my best friend shot me in the head. Instead, I was walking around an empty street in Oxford, a roguish fantasy outlaw sent to recover an ancient tome of unspeakable knowledge from the clutches of some evil empire.

It turns out there was something else I wanted: pity. I sought reaction, acknowledgment. I sought shock value. *Something.* There was a handful of us in the class, maybe fifteen—at most, only two knew what had happened. The others asked me, from what they could see under my Timberwolves knit hat, why I shaved my head. Did I lose a bet or something? To this day, most of the students from my graduating class have no idea I was shot on April 7, 2017.

PROTOCOL

It's difficult to separate *what* happened and *where* it happened. It happened at a private institution beholden to policies set in place to mitigate liability and legal risks. Inevitably, there was always going to be a certain abrasiveness between my legal complaint and their legal position. In a sense, they weren't responsible for what had happened; shootings happen on campus, all too often, even when there are (supposedly) strict bans of firearms on campus. But in another more personal sense, the University made it impossible for me to truly pardon them. There are legal restraints that inhibit anyone involved in a lawsuit from acting like a human being; I can live with that, I suppose. However, the University afforded Mark a kind of grace they did not extend to me. There would have been space for reconciliation between the University and me, had they taken a less cynical and more ethical course of action. But they abandoned me by the wayside, and in doing so, smothered dialogue about gun violence that is vital and necessary.

What did they do instead? They covered their asses. First: they ran with Mark's version of events. They never challenged his story or investigated its gaps and inconsistencies. If that story was foolproof, they wouldn't have had to forge the Public Safety report—which is exactly what they did. They know their Public Safety officer neglected to examine the apartment despite alarm, smoke, blood, and the smell of burning. I've seen more rigorous searches by Public Safety officers looking for a bottle of Ron Diaz Spiced Rum. (It was found in some ductwork, hidden there by someone on my floor freshman year.)

Second: they followed protocol by sending a mass text alerting students and faculty that a gun had discharged on campus. They did not, however, follow up this diligence with decency. They did not call my emergency contact (my mother). They did not fill her in on every known detail (the hospital where I was admitted, that I wasn't dead). They did take the time to post on Facebook, disclosing that a student was injured. They played down the severity of this injury, focusing instead on the health of the school in general: yes, the sanctity of the school had been shaken, but rest assured, students, that if anyone needs any counseling, on-campus services are available to you. This was the only social media post about the shooting. There was no further communication in any form to the student body or to the public. No details. No teachable moment. Not even any thoughts and prayers.

Third: the University took meetings. The president of the University met with Mark. They did not meet with me or my mother. Instead, they issued us a defensive and pushy statement, basically a *hell no*: our med pay insurance policy only goes into effect upon death. *Death.* They had no obligation to provide financial help with either medical expenses or tuition, even though it happened on campus. Might they have done something out of charitable spirit? Waiving tuition, an institutional donation, community fundraising? Could they have at the least sent me a legally vetted note of apology? No. Any of this would have made them look negligent and uncaring, which they were.

GRADUATION

Nearing the end of the academic year, I went back on campus for what felt like the first time since the shooting to pick up my tassel and honors medal for graduation. Being there hit different during the light of day, when the University resembled its truest self. The cycles of movement, a high-functioning atmosphere, tons and tons of people with someplace to be. There was not much room for the fantasy that imbued my campus walks to class. Just the cold, hard facts.

It was wet out. The air smelled like a rainy Sunday plus candied almonds plus mildew and lo-fi underground hip-hop—a perfume I love but whose name I don't know. Mom and I didn't want to pay the school three dollars for underground parking, the same garage that is directly below where I used to live, the same garage where Mark stashed his guns, so we wasted ten minutes cruising around for a free spot on the street.

We found one near some housing being rented out by university students. On a driveway, no more than twenty feet away: a navy-blue sedan. Mark's car.

I knew the license plate by heart; we had taken it road-tripping to his cabin up north, driven it during our late-night excursions for cheap food. It took a minute to really sink in—this was *Mark's car*. We had entered the newly cursed grounds of the shooting. Where it happened, who did it, and who it happened to, all within one hundred yards of each other once again. Surrounded by these landmarks, the cruel, chaotic, residual energy of that night was palpable.

I held an umbrella in one hand and grabbed Mom's shoulder with the other as we crossed the street to official school property. In recovery, my walks had been minimal. Bed to bathroom to couch and back to bed. This felt long; too much.

Mom asked how I was doing once we hit the grass, and I gestured so-so with a teetering hand. I could throw a rock at my old window if I wanted to. I kind of wanted to.

We passed the wooden bench where I officially asked Anna to go out with me on April 6, 2014; it had been an otherwise clear, ordinary spring day. Mark, Keith, and the rest of our friends had cheered me on from a nearby bush. Doing a terrible job of hiding, they added a sketch comedy quirkiness to my first-ever romantic escapade.

Think of all my good memories like this: they're at a party, mingling, toasting, joking, dancing, having an intimate conversation here, a serious one over there, casual chitchat all around, romance in certain corners. Then the memory of getting shot arrives. The music cuts. The PA system emits white noise, like in a paranormal investigation show, overwhelming the room with fear and static and the voice of the Ghost of April 7:

"MARK IS IN THE HALLWAY, WITH ONE HAND OVER HIS MOUTH, THE OTHER HOLDING A GUN. YOU ARE SENT TO THE GROUND, SUDDENLY. YOU THINK IT IS A NUCLEAR BOMB, STUPID BOY."

What used to feel sacred now feels haunted.

While navigating the quad with Mom, I spotted an acquaintance; we'd taken a few classes together over the years. I pulled my knit hat down, nearly over my eyes, wanting nothing more than for him to not recognize me. I didn't want anyone to see me like this, struggling to walk, holding onto Mom. I was sad and upset, which made me sadder and more upset. How dare my feelings be so predictable?

EXPELLED

Home for a few days, still trying to readjust to the world of the living. Anna calls. I put it on speaker and hold the phone very far away from my head.

"I just saw Mark," Anna says. "I was moving things from my apartment to my car and ran into him on the sidewalk; just off campus, by the SuperAmerica."

After the shooting, Anna decided to commute from home to school for the remainder of the semester. She didn't like passing the building where we first met. Freshman year, we had found ourselves in the same English class, Monsters: In Me and Around Me, where we studied books about vampires, reanimated corpses, and Nazis, trying to deduce what makes someone or something monstrous. The room was paired off on the first day. Anna and I were both number eight, and she waved awkwardly across a row of computers. I pulled a chair out for her to sit. The icebreaker was to talk about our favorite villains.

When she tells me she's seen Mark again, I'm unsure what to say that's of any substance. "Oh."

"He said he's expelled from school. And then he asked if he could hug me."

"Oh," I say again. If I were her, I would have ignored him outright, his privileges to approach me, revoked. There are two sides now: the shooter, and the shot. Like warring families in a Shakespearean drama. A line has been drawn.

"I hugged him, and he apologized," Anna says. "He said he will never be able to look any of us in eye ever again."

"Uh huh," I say. Can't blame him there. When everyone should be picking sides, here's Anna, extending the olive branch. She got the apology I never did.

"I couldn't look him in the eye either," Anna says. "I didn't know if I should hide in the parking garage or say something. We were good friends too, you know."

She's right. They were friends, independent of me. I should have no objections about a hug in the power of a moment. It just seems too soon. The gift of Anna's forgiveness, to me, is something Mark in no way has earned.

"How do you feel?" she asks.

"I have a headache." An easy workaround. An obvious default. How could I confront these things when I couldn't even confront subtracting seven from one hundred more than twice?

"About me running into Mark." Anna forces my hand.

"I'm glad no one is pressing charges," I say, maintaining my diplomatic stance. Whatever trouble is in store for Mark, I will not be the reason—I will not add vengeance to the situation. I am the victim. I am not the aggressor.

"I'm glad he got expelled though." My stance didn't mean there shouldn't be commensurate punishment, accountability. Expulsion was a start. A little closure hors d'oeuvre; though, like most appetizers, it was short lived.

"Yeah. I'm sorry I hugged him. I kind of regret it now," Anna says.

"No worries, for real." I mean it.

After we hang up, I tell Mom that Mark got expelled.

"I don't like it," she says. "He is already over it. He's back to his normal life. There needs to be more consequences. You will be different forever."

I remind her it was a freak accident. That perhaps Mark is more complex than his actions on April 7, trying to convince myself of the same. He may not have pages of residual symptoms, but maybe a few paragraphs of remorse.

She shakes her head, fanning down my plea with a firm and halting hand gesture that asks, *But which one of you got shot?*

GRADUATION II

The class of 2017 fills the university gymnasium, but there is at least one exception: Mark is not here. Which means I am. Being back makes my stomach feel like I hopped the fence into a No Trespassing zone. The fuzzy churn of my perceived excommunication, combined with a general unease. Still, I want to close the loop on school. This ritual might just do the trick. I think I've earned it, in the least.

It is raining, so the ceremony has been moved indoors. The gym has a Jumbotron. The person reading the names pronounces nothing right, including my name. People are mad. But I am dressed and ready to walk these steps and have made sure to test how the cap rubs up against my wound so I can angle it in such a way as to mitigate pain. The University had given me as many tickets as I needed for graduation, so all my family members could be there.

When called, I walk as straight as I can. I do not slip on the short, bleacher-like temporary staircase. Onstage, I do not tumble and make a scene. But I wonder, as I'm handed a proxy envelope (diploma coming soon, notwithstanding parking tickets or late fees), if this person shaking my hand knows who I am, that I was the one who was shot on campus two months ago.

I had hopes that the University president would pull me aside, in private, and formally apologize today. Mom wanted them to announce it during the ceremony, to thunderous applause, that I had made it. But neither happened. I don't feel welcome here. I feel like a dirty little secret. Should I wink?

I'm moved along, standing now on the photographer's mark on the stage floor. I'm asked to smile. Hurry, please—next!

LITIGATION

The ambulance ride, emergency room visit, intensive care, anesthesia, surgery, and eight-day recovery stay at the hospital—after some insurance—cost about $80,000, some of which was waived when Mom told the billing department I was a broke college kid with insurmountable student loan debt. Primary care, neurology clinics, talk therapy, EMDR therapy, physical therapy, occupational therapy, headache specialists, and surgery checkups totaled roughly $20,000. I had insurance for most of the initial care, then was uninsured later on. With everything tallied, the last line on the ledger was still a daunting $60,000. To no one's surprise, we did not have that kind of money lying around.

Each time Mom set up an out-of-pocket payment plan to fend off being sent to collections, I died a little inside. She was worried about my credit. I was worried about her retirement. Prior to any kind of formal lawsuit, we were financially responsible for it all.

Two or three weeks after the accident, a lawyer pulled up to the house in a silver BMW and gave us his spiel. One of Mom's coworkers recommended him. He was in his midforties and had cool rings, a stylish navy suit, a dark brown crew cut completely immobilized by hair gel with added shine, and suave, angular features that on a billboard (though he's far too classy for that) would suggest: *I'm ethical but willing to be ballsy*. Simply put, he looked like he won a lot of cases.

The whole experience was not unlike those sport-recruitment scenes in movies, where a coach or agent tries to convince the star player and their mom to join the team. It was the only time in my life I've ever felt like a child prodigy. His spiel: he knew my life would never be the same, knew no amount of money would make what happened okay, knew this was harrowing for me and my family, and therefore his mission was to get me what I was owed.

Finally, someone who got it. Someone on our side. He understood the stakes.

I signed my name on a line that gave him 33.3 percent of whatever amount we ended up with. With that, I had a lawyer.

The lawyer investigated things and advised it wasn't in our best interest to sue the University. I didn't get an in-depth reason at the time, but legal negligence is not even remotely the same as plain old accountability. (The University will most likely never take a hit from this. Largely still a mystery—at best—April 7 was a blip on their radar. Admissions are higher than ever. The donations for new, technologically advanced student centers keep pouring in.)

Accountability in my case was elusive. Blame was at the foot of the University and their Public Safety department, sure, but let's zoom out. Without the gun lobby and the corporate influence of gun manufacturers and the craven legislators who happily do their bidding, there wouldn't be, as of this writing, 393 million guns in a country of 326 million people, not even including military or law enforcement service weapons.[1] The blame should go around but only one person was stupid or careless enough to pull the trigger.

Our strategy was to focus all efforts on Mark. Mark had promised he would pay for everything; this, however, was right after he shot me, while he was in a state of mind that you might not call right. And while, yes, his parents were shouldering the responsibility of payment, they weren't generously writing checks. A typical homeowner's insurance policy includes coverage for personal liability claims, as theirs did: any money awarded to me would come directly from the insurance company. And they had plenty of coverage. The court papers would list Mark as the defendant, but in actuality it was me versus a billion-dollar corporation.

All things considered, I figured this shouldn't take long. It's a cut-and-dry personal injury settlement. Bullet, walls, head—case closed. We should be popping corks by the end of the summer. I did not, could not, understand how much of my life this process would take, on top of the injury itself. I greatly underestimated the cruelty built into the business model of insurance companies. The lengths they went to torment me felt exceptional, personal.

After the lawyer left, David pulled me aside.

"So, any chance there will be a trial?" he asked.

A fair question, but I got mad, flickering him looks of bitterness, disgust. The threat of a trial was real, but it was as if David asked, "So, any chance Mark doesn't want to help?" Does he, in fact, want to fight this lawsuit, which in essence would be salt in the wound? Basically: Do you think that Mark is a bad guy?

I told David no, all snarky and ornery. In truth, I knew how little control Mark had over this whole settlement thing; ultimately, his leverage was minuscule at most. But he had promised, I thought. He wants this to go just as smooth as I do. I know it. He was my friend.

I was informed that during this process that I wasn't allowed to talk to Mark, and that he wasn't allowed to talk to me. I had no idea if he wanted to.

PROOF

Mark's insurance company requires a picture of my crater and scar for proof, which is something I don't understand at the time. I make several attempts, feeling increasingly exposed, as if they had demanded dick pics as part of some blackmail scheme.

"You don't have to cut your hair, just part it if you can. Make sure we can see everything," read their detailed, step-by-step instructions.

I wait until Mom leaves for work, stand in the middle of the kitchen, and take about twenty photos. I hold a clump of hair like a paintbrush above the long pink fleshy line along my scalp. It feeds into the crater the way a river feeds a lake, then continues as a river on the other side.

It's hard to take photos of the top of your head with one hand. I can't get the correct angle so I go to the bathroom, assuming the mirror will help somehow and take twenty more photos. I'm crying in the final eight or nine, but the shots don't capture anything below the forehead.

BLAME

I didn't have to frantically imagine Mark's backstory, his reasons, his problems. I was his best friend. I sympathized with him where others could not, forgave him where others could not. This made hatred a pretty tall order.

But after the shooting there were times, mostly late at night, when I couldn't help but imagine him as this pompous asshole, gleefully going about his everyday business, who never paid me any mind and regretted nothing.

Caught in the infinite in-between that bloomed after the accident, it was painful to think of Mark in any regard, friend or foe. Lucky for him (or me?), he had a proxy: his insurance company. They proved to be a reliable punching bag, the only truly shitty party with zero redeeming qualities. I'd love to complicate them with layers or shades of gray, but they are as old-school baddie as it gets, and they took the brunt of the fall: all my stray emotions, all my anger, all of it.

I decided that once we settled, I would forget all about Mark. I would forget about the University and Public Safety. I would forget about America's Gun Problem. I would no longer worry about who to blame. Money would check that box, fill that void.

I would move on, morally superior and revitalized.

I would move on.

PARANOIA

Thirty days since the shooting. I've become an avid window-watcher from beneath the sheets. I check things and keep track. I check the outside world at least fifteen times every hour. I'm sure it's not healthy, but checking feels good, and that reinforces the urge to check. It's like waiting for a package—not for something I ordered, but rather some*one* who will abduct and imprison me, confine me to a torture facility, and cause me great bodily harm. Waterboarding, pendulums, blow torches, bomb collars. Checking feels good. I am on alert. I'm through with surprises.

Mom and David's place is in a new development; that is, it is still developing, which means there is plenty to check and track. There are cars, vans, trucks, machines, and construction workers, always in motion, always doing something related to building houses in bulk. There is surveying equipment out at the ends of driveways, as if for sale, also checking and tracking things, same as me. There is dirt and orange and cones and constant rhythmic pounding, like a Black Sabbath song. The difference is that I like Black Sabbath.

As I write this, there is a red truck parked across the street. I assume it's the neighbor's, but I never see anyone get in or out of it. The headlights are on, though they weren't a minute ago. That sedan farther down the road—someone is in the passenger seat, watching me watch them. A branded utility vehicle under the streetlight has moved closer to our house, if only by a foot or so. It also has a different logo than yesterday. That person, there—who in their right mind is walking their dog right now amid all this construction? It is almost dark. On second thought, it's midday, so it's almost, almost dark. Why are they so close to our curb? I feel like I'm under house arrest.

Everyone seems to be on the phone, looking at their phones, pointing their cameras toward me and the house. There are people pointing, with serious expressions, tasked with some reconnaissance mission against me. They are paid to blend in as construction workers, or a new cable company, but are really taking stock of my well-being, wanting to take me to their torture facility for questioning and/or great bodily harm. Cages, sleep deprivation, eye gouging, and finger removal.

It might sound like I'm paranoid, but my lawyer says it is not uncommon for insurance companies to investigate victims in personal injury cases. Some checking and tracking of their own. It is a real job for real people. These agents get paid to monitor me and assess my settlement numbers. They are paid to ensure I'm not lying, maybe even paid on a commission basis, so there's incentive to bend evidence. They are reporting to a scary, terrible man in charge, who I imagine walks with a cane and still smokes indoors at the secret torture facility even though smoking indoors there is sort of frowned upon, but he's the boss so everybody lets it go. Nobody with kids of their own could spy on other people's children, I think. If they do have kids, these settlement agents, I bet their kids hate them. I have a lot of time to think about these things.

My lawyer tells me to be wary. Try not to share too much online. I get the itch to change my name and create burner accounts. He says anything and everything can and will be used against me. Things I could do to better myself, to heal myself, things that would make me feel wholesome—a walk outside, meeting up for coffee with an old friend, applying for a job, uploading a video of me playing guitar to YouTube, sharing some writing on Twitter—these things are now counterevidence to my injury. I want to get better. Better than before, even. But it is not in my best legal interest to get better. I'm incentivized to not even try.

At night, I imagine they use a thermal imaging scanner to watch me sleep. The guy in the passenger seat of the sedan watches my breath pass, as if I'm a human fog machine. He monitors the occasional fart. They've rigged the ceiling fan above me to drop but they don't know I'm on to them, not yet. I'm going to be strategic about it. One of them takes a break at four in the morning, checks his phone, his OkCupid page. I'd wait for the glow of his phone screen to reveal his face and then point from my window directly at him. He'd hurriedly strap his seatbelt on, think, *Oh shit, I've been made*, and then squeal away leaving tire marks. I would win, with my eagle eye.

I smell my sweat soaking into Mom's brand-new sheets. It is an odd smell, residue from the manufacturing process mixed with tart, stressful discharge, creating a chlorine-vinegar-anxiety solution. It's a smell that won't leave me alone throughout recovery. I can call upon it still. The sheets are stiff with factory creases. I can't get comfortable, stirring in excess fabric. My head is throbbing. My implant wants out. In fear of clogged pores and breakouts, I force myself up to rinse off.

There are phantom sirens in the shower water. I leave it running and investigate in my towel. Something changed when I saw my name in the news. It is messing with me.

New worries emerge daily. I know technically what they are. I know the science, the case studies, the DSM definitions. But I can't rationalize why I'm now so afraid of a piece of paper being slid under a door. The sound of unexpected knocking. The ring of a doorbell. Why am I so afraid of people holding clipboards on TV? Black Cadillac Escalades? I throw away an apple with mysterious red streaks that I assume is poisonous. Mom shrugs but doesn't stop me.

Certain worries are blunter than others. I'm afraid of people standing behind me within shooting distance. I'm afraid of fire detectors. Their dumb presence, their tense potential to sound off at any moment, especially before bed. I watch the LED sensors blink: green, green, red, trying to anticipate the color, so sure I caught a chirp. Mom forgets garlic bread in the oven, and I'm a gray blob, stripped of function and responsibility, cupping my hands over my ears in acute panic. Where are the cops? Why is no one helping me?

As my brain heals, as I slowly recover my wits, just as the pain becomes bearable, hypervigilance and paranoia creep in, take over, unwanted houseguests that slowly poison my food and take pictures of me as I sleep.

The neighbor's truck is gone again.

BLUES

When I was nine or ten, I made it my duty to play guitar for all the maintenance workers Mom hired for house projects. I was spoiled with a huge music room in the basement, full of posters, guitar paraphernalia, and a four-disk CD player to jam along to. I made custom playlists and would turn up the master volume on my amp in incremental nudges until I was positive everyone could hear as I played along. If you are installing cable or renovating the kitchen, here are some tunes while you work. Putting on an audible showcase, doing them a favor, really. In no way obnoxious. Not to brag, but I was easily the best nine or ten-year-old blues guitarist on the block.

I'm double-jointed in my middle finger on my left hand. As a kid, I considered that to be a guitar superpower, predisposing me to quickness and finger strength and an ability to bend strings in unconventional ways with soulful precision. Plus, I have synesthesia. I didn't know that word at the time; I just knew I could see color on the fretboard when playing in different keys. My hearing sense is paired with my seeing sense. Each key has a distinct color and relates to music theory in a cool way.

That day, I was probably playing along to a Cream tune in C, which makes certain segments of the fretboard glow like desert sand gold. Shifting between major and minor scales is like changing where the sun is in the sky.

I was born to play guitar, I thought.

The man painting our entranceway asked to shake my hand as I emerged from the basement in need of a fruit snack.

"Wow, I gotta do this before you're famous!" he said.

I felt electrified, like the wires powering my would-be marquee: Bulletproof Paul and the Drywalls, Tonight Only, Sold Out.

After the shooting, I didn't touch a guitar until Mom and David had a guy over to fix the floors. I'm upstairs in the loft with blankets taped over all the windows, the whole space like the inside of an eyelid facing the sun, the idea of a womb, perhaps, when I hear the noise downstairs. Leaky pipe. Warped wood. I dig out an amp from a moving box. I lift the hinges on a guitar case Anna brought back from school. Master volume nudged incrementally as bravado increases. Until I'm sure everyone can hear it.

My fingertips miss their callouses. I hadn't realized how much I craved the feel of wrapped nickel strings reshaping the skin. Press, fret, bend: all sexy, dirty words to me now.

Yes, it's too loud. Of course it hurts. But Guitar Paul is a Blues Legend. He is heart and soul. He bites my lip. He throws my head back and sings:

Well, it was a Friday when my best friend shot me down.

Yeah! It was a Friday when my best friend shot me down.

Just like old times, Mom comes upstairs and freaks out, threatens to pull the plug, take everything away. I plead my case. She grants me fifteen more minutes. Cut the volume in half, then half of half.

The colors are gone for now—the synesthesia seems to be gone, which is kind of sad. Still double-jointed, so I got that going for me. My fretting hand is sweaty as I play. I'm trying to go faster than usual. Testing my ability. I know what I want to play, but the transmission from brain to hand isn't quite there. I'm clunky. Out of shape. Missing some notes, falling off the binding at times. But before long, I settle in and gain some confidence.

Improvising on guitar recycles my mind's neuroses. I fear the room is bugged, or that a settlement agent is outside with a decibel meter, so I play quick muted notes, lost arpeggios. I lean into the pain, now head and fingers, and let the thickest string ring out while I bend two notes in tandem, making them clash, the good dissonance. The stuff that sounds wrong on purpose.

I get my frustration out. Big chords, powerful strums. I think about how Mark and I used to play together. The blues reaches its peak at heartbreak.

I emerge from the loft in need of Tylenol. No handshake this time; the floor guy is out getting something from his van.

I wonder if he's heard about me on the news.

VIDEO GAME

Another day confined to the loft. I'm slung over on the floor like a wind-blown scarecrow. Mom and David are yelling at each other downstairs. I hold my breath and listen to the argument run its course like a fever. It reminds me of my parents on their way to divorce.

Next to the TV sits *BioShock 2* in its flashy metallic case. Anna bought me the collector's edition for my birthday last year, all remastered and prettier now. Anna's dream life would be living in the Mediterranean, windows open and playing video games endlessly in a walkout basement.

Though it is a trilogy, I'd somehow missed the second game. I figure now is as good a time as any to connect the dots—my schedule is pretty open. I attach the necessary wires to their corresponding inputs and out-puts and outlets, hoping to use nostalgia like medicine. Anything to keep me in my own mind. I'll take it even if it hurts.

Within minutes, past some loading screens and calibrations, I am somewhere beneath the Atlantic Ocean in the hedonistic ruins of an underwater city. Set in 1958, there is a haunting doo-wop soundscape, one that is stylistically correct for the game's mood and its juxtaposition of violence and utopia.

I've become a mutated person in an oversized, old-fashioned deep-sea diving suit. It is a marvelous suit, the classic bubble helmet with a cluster of warm, glowing spheres where my eyes would be. There is a brushed metal oxygen tank on my back that has a faded red valve. I'm equipped with matching boots and gloves, looking meticulously crafted out of leather and copper. Where my right arm should be is instead a titanic industrial drill.

When the city was in its prime, these creatures were originally designed to keep everything in the city running smoothly and fix whatever needed repair. Now, their drills are used for devastating melees. I'm tasked with keeping my toddler-aged daughter safe.

The TV distorts as water pours from certain parts of the environment, causing everything to ripple in realtime as if I were really in the helmet. This feeling of total immersion throws me for a loop. I look at a pillow on the floor next to me to center myself again. The front of my brain feels heavy. I can almost feel my neurons firing, my motor working. After a few hard blinks, I successfully clear my slate and carry on.

Enemies go after my daughter. They lure her into a corner. They surround her. I thunder over to intervene, clunky posture and all. I am heavy. I am mean. I am blunt. I am cold. I am brutish. And I care a lot about this little girl—*my* little girl.

The enemies open fire. Bullets are ricocheting off my diving suit. I go ballistic with the drill, piercing through torsos with morbid torque. The little girl's survival is reliant upon my survival. Therefore, this violence is justified, but I cannot bring myself to shoot at the head. I aim for the chest. I set a moral standard for how to destroy the pixels onscreen.

One enemy throws a powerful orb at me. The rules of the game are such that it puts me in a hypnotic trance when it hits. They can now control my actions with their voice. My daughter is crying. She wants desperately to help and wants desperately not to see me hurt.

The enemy tells me to kneel, and I do. They tell me to remove my helmet, and I do. They tell me to take their pistol, and I do. They tell me to place it against my head, and I do. They tell me to pull the trigger. My daughter screams. I pull the trigger.

The screen goes black. My controller hits the floor.

I massage the sheet of skin covering my crater. It's pulled taut, as thin as the skin of an apple.

In the game, I learn that ten years have passed since that incident. Weeks have passed since mine. My avatar—Diving Suit Dude as I call him—wakes up in the exact same place as he got shot, slow to rise but alive.

I want to cheer him on. We did it, Diving Suit Dude; we will have our issues, but we did it! We are a slurry of post-traumatic stress disorder and a traumatic brain injury, each diagnosis feeding and reinforcing the other. We are the perfect storm of a short-circuiting supercomputer disguised as ground beef molded into a fist. We are alike in the most improbable way. We have quests and objectives and people who care about us.

I call Anna, put it on speaker, and hold the phone very far away from my head. *What a coincidence. No, I haven't played it until now, this is my first time. Isn't that just strange. The timing of it all, the plot so far. Ridiculous, I know.*

MULTIVERSE

Whenever Mom gets really stressed, a cold sore forms right below her nostril in the middle of her Cupid's bow. I noticed it when I was first at the hospital after the shooting and again yesterday but still haven't said anything. I have been in her house for four weeks.

She is in the back seat of the Chrysler, croaking nonsense to my sister Krystin's infant daughter, Alli. Mom's got puffy eyes and Alli is contorting all weird. I can tell little sleep was had last night.

I'm in the passenger seat and will be for at least another two months. The angsty teen again. Reliant on my family for rides. Mom's singing the melody of "Ba Ba Black Sheep" but with doo's in exchange for the traditional folk lyrics. It's going on too long. I'm so out of it I can't tell her to quit. As my caregiver for the past few weeks, witness to all I've suffered, every affliction and hardship, I assumed she would know better.

Krystin is behind the wheel with her cell phone's GPS open in her lap. I am sensitive to light and sound, was told these are common symptoms in my uncommon circumstance. I pull my knit hat over my head and look through the stitching's pores. Focusing on one hole helps with the overstimulation. Each hole is a little different. I pretend it's like the sponge theory of the multiverse, that each hole allows me to glimpse entirely different worlds.

My mother, grief-stricken, sulks, mourning the loss of my twinkle: some inherent, jovial quality she claims I used to have that lent itself to my good-natured spirit and overall fun-loving, witty disposition. She is worried on my behalf about residual symptoms: poor sleep, seizures, post-traumatic stress, and mental fatigue. She knows I'll never really be me again. She has said this—to my face—on multiple occasions.

I'm more worried about what I'll miss out on in life. Roller coasters, holding my breath underwater, a chance to date Emilia Clarke. I'm worried the injury took a few years off, too, that I'm going to die younger, sooner. I thought that perhaps something weird would change, maybe for the better. Like I'd never have to sneeze again. Or that I could suddenly speak Japanese. Stuff like that happens with head injuries. Not mine. Any positives that come out of this, I'll have to earn the hard way.

We get off at our exit. The ride was quicker than expected. I peer out into a universe of my choosing from within my knit hat. A light beam glares through as I pick the world where I'm not getting nineteen staples removed from my head today.

STAPLES

The surgeon who performed my craniotomy enters the examination room. He is wearing a cool vest with fashionable leather shoes. Mom and I are both pleased with how nice he looks. Until now, we've only ever seen him in plain, sanitary garb. His taste in street clothes reminds me of Mark. If Mark was wearing clothes, which wasn't a common occurrence, at least not in our apartment, he made sure to look sharp. Junior year, he and I decided to dress up to class once per week. Donning blazers, suspenders, and ties, sometimes straight, sometimes bow. Our name for it, pure genius: Fancy Fridays.

The surgeon brings up my CT scan pictures from April 7 and compares them to the ones just taken this afternoon. He tells me I'm the only person he's talked to who's been shot in the head. Most people don't talk after something like that, he says. Most people die.

"In fact," he says, "if the bullet hit an inch higher, you would have been paralyzed from the waist down. If it had hit an inch lower, you wouldn't have made it at all."

I'm squeamish, so I rub the dry skin off my lips to distract me. It rolls up over itself like a brand-new poster. My surgeon goes on to tell me that people have had life-altering concussions from simply getting punched in the face.

"You got shot," he says, as if I had forgotten, "and you will have concussion-like symptoms, tenfold." He says new residuals could emerge years from now.

I think about all the things that could have happened while a nurse rubs iodine over my incision, preparing to clip out the staples. For all intents and purposes, the instrument used is almost no different from a staple remover found in any junk drawer. It feels like I'm getting poked by a thumbtack, nineteen times.

If I hadn't leaned over, I would have been shot in the stomach. Which would have had its own unique problems. More blood, more immediate complications.

I imagine every possible outcome branching off into its own space in the multiverse. As soon as the firearm discharged, tons of successional states of being. A different wound with infinite repetition. Wounds covering my entire body. There are worlds where the bullet misses, although in others it goes through an eye. That's one of the more gruesome ones, along with the throat. I think about the throat a lot, playing out little three-second blips of scene.

I tuck my forehead in the crook of my elbow as if sleeping at a stand-up desk.

I'm grabbing and slipping at my neck, not really trying to stop the bleeding, just trying to figure out what's going on.

Through the heart, I do that tough-guy shoulder shimmy like a Western movie death.

There are kneecappings and arm grazes. Penetrations through my shins and hands. There is one where my cheekbone shatters like a teacup thrown against a wall, and one where my teeth are shot out like a clown in a carnival game. I swallow the bullets with a cartoon gulp.

On the way home, I call Anna on speaker, holding the phone very far away from my head. She is happy to hear my voice, happy to hear that the staple removal hurt less than I expected. She says there are still times when she thinks I died on April 7, that people are putting on an elaborate facade that I survived for her sake. When I text her, it's actually one of my sisters pretending to be me. They will keep this up as long as possible. So Anna doesn't go do something stupid.

THERAPY

I start talk therapy about a month after the shooting. Aside from the lone session I was court-ordered to have after my parents divorced, where I sort of *Good Will Hunting*'d the poor guy, saying nothing of substance so I wouldn't have to come back, this was my first meaningful one-on-one with a therapist. The office is an old repurposed Victorian mansion. The little goth inside me approves. My therapist's name is Jim. Jim is bald and reveals he, too, had an accident that resulted in a traumatic brain injury.

"As you can see." He points to an M-shaped indent on top of his head.

"Mine is a crater," I say.

I don't ask how his TBI happened. And he doesn't explain.

I stumble through my spiel all antsy as always, naming off every misdeed, rapid fire, in whatever order it happens to pop up in my head.

Jim takes a minute and mentions he may have read something about me in the paper.

Then Jim says the brain likes to compartmentalize things into beginnings, middles, and ends. He said I've been homing in on the end, but I need to start constructing the rest of what happened that day—before the shooting—to manifest an integration.

"Integration," I say, echoing him. It sounds impressive, but nothing like the word *closure*.

"That way, when you think about the shooting before bed one night, you have a plan in place, and can easily switch to what you ate for breakfast or what the weather was like that day, for example. Preparation is key with trauma. Know what you're going to think about ahead of time."

"Preparation," I echo, skeptical. How was thinking back to my Frosted Flakes or the springtime humidity going to combat intrusive thoughts? Isn't that masking the real issue?

I'm willing to try most anything once, except here's the wrinkle: at this point, sitting in Jim's office, I don't remember *anything* about April 7 before the shooting.

I didn't have class on Fridays, so I probably slept in. I was on the verge of getting sick; I remember not wanting to go to the doctor. There is a selfie saved on my phone from that morning although I don't remember taking it: me, in bed, a dazed shell of myself, with tissue plugs in my nose that I must've inserted to dam off an excess of runny mucus. I used a filter that superimposed a dinosaur costume on my body like I was some minor league baseball mascot. Was it overcast outside? Drizzling? The following nine hours were a complete blur of our living room, that forest green sofa. Did I just mope around with Mark? Play video games? I found a save file of *The Witcher 3* that dates 12:34 p.m. April 7, 2017. We probably did just hang out. We did that often. Zero memory of this. Seeing this time stamp knocked the wind out of me. I even cried a little. I played video games until what? Until I felt guilted into homework? What did I eat? Did I even eat? Did I ever change out of my pajamas? I know I never left the apartment until I was carried out by gurney.

Don't think about the gurney.

I have a feeling this will be a problem.

I tell Jim that I can't remember anything else about April 7. "Is that a problem?" I ask.

"The day before works as well," Jim said.

The day before was sunny, maybe a little breezy. I went on a walk with Anna. It was our three-year anniversary. We walked to the Tea Garden, located a short jaunt away from school. We bought each other bubble tea; I paid for hers, she paid for mine. We thought that was a funny idea. We sat on backless barstools, precast seats form-fitted like a child's swing at a playground. I recall being fascinated by the machine that sealed a film top onto each cup. I nudged Anna whenever it sprang into action. We had a great view.

I ordered watermelon-strawberry. Anna got cherry-kiwi. We both selected a green tea base, with tapioca pearls.

"Smile!" she said.

"You know I hate taking pictures in public."

"It's our three-year."

"Fine. No redoes if it's bad."

"I'll look good no matter what."

"True," I said.

Knocking me off my cloud, Jim asks me what I want out of these therapy sessions. What do I want? I want closure for something that is still a scabbing wound on the top of my head. Honestly, I just want to get better. I consider establishing a SMART goal for the rest of my life, like we did in grade school, something Specific, Measurable, Attainable, Relevant, and Time-based.

I look around the room. I like this room. It feels alive, as if there are billions of little microorganisms in the ceiling. Active cultures of the good bacteria. Like in yogurt. I like that everything feels like it is covered in moss.

The silence grows heavy. I haven't answered.

"For instance," Jim prompts me, "one might want the outcome to transcend the incident itself in the long run. Sort of in spite of what happened."

"Yes," I say. "That's a good one."

He smiles. Then he asks about Mark and my feelings toward him.

I say, "Mostly, I'm just sad."

"Why is that?"

"I really liked him," I say.

"What do you hope he feels?"

I picture Mark unceremoniously opening his school-issued wooden safe, gun and ammunition hidden away like pornography. He pulls out a molded case and places it on his dresser. After releasing the latches, he cleans his gun with a microfiber cloth stained with lubricating oils. Maybe there is a song stuck in his head, or maybe he is thinking of *John Wick*, *Bad Boys*, *The Godfather*—something gives him the itch to pull. He selects a target, the wall, toward me and the rest of our apartment, he maybe even closes an eye, and he turns his gun to the side for style points, to show he's done this plenty of times before. He knows it's wrong and shoots anyway. Whether he knew it or not, he pointed a gun at me, his best friend, and, whether he intended to or not, pulled the trigger.

"I hope that he's perhaps more risk averse now?" I think I sound dumb but Jim reassures me I don't. "Maybe more empathetic? Punctual? Trustworthy?"

"Do you see yourself ever hanging out with him again? Meeting up?" he prompts, twirling a pen by his ear as if it were a laser pointer toying with some imaginary cat behind me.

"I'm not sure," I say.

"How do you think you would react if you saw him?" Jim asks.

"I would be terrified."

COFFEE

My sister Alyssa comes by the house one day and makes a suggestion. Why don't we go grab a coffee, stretch your legs?

I'm worried about reintroducing caffeine to my brain after a TBI. I have no evidence to support this hesitation. Just thinking of the substance not as coffee but as a chemical makes me nervous. On the other hand, seeing natural things, being outside, speeds up the recovery process, my surgeon says. I should get out and walk. Provided I go properly equipped.

I am the biggest sucker for those "gear up" scenes in every spy or superhero movie. I love watching characters don their costumes and collect their gadgets, hearing the satisfying clicks of each meticulous piece fitting together perfectly, every tie, zip, buckle, and tuck. Something about small mechanical objects with a specific purpose.

Ever since I was little, I've adored putting on layered clothing for a similar reason. It's woven armor, a personal, incognito super-suit. Tube socks under joggers and jeans. T-shirts under button-down collared long sleeves, crew neck sweaters, and hooded zip-ups. Things kick up a notch when it gets cold out in home sweet Minnesnowta. And does it ever get cold. Every winter, I bust out my coat with insulation like peppered tinfoil, the latest tech, though it's currently stowed away in a mudroom closet until absolutely necessary. Is this my kink?

My knit hat may not have retractable razor blades, nor my sunglasses any lasers or augmented reality capabilities, but I need them. Anything to make me feel like a Jedi or Power Ranger again.

And yet today, post-shooting, even an old pair of basketball shoes feel foreign, awkward, heavy, as I use all my strength to climb into Alyssa's car.

We head to an artsy Main Street coffee shop, the only non-chain establishment for miles. No street parking, so we find a garage. More walking. Though I'm fifteen pounds underweight (but slowly gaining, hungrier than ever, with two, sometimes three servings of dinner per night), pallid, gangly, phantom-like, purple bags with swirls of pink and blue beneath my eyes, limping like I have a broken femur—I blend in here more than ever. An emerging patron saint of the basket-case lifestyle. Especially with the clothing. A winter hat in spring. Mistaken as too cool to care about health or longevity. Don't be fooled. I care too much now.

Favoring one leg, avoiding a certain heel-toe combination, I stumble into crosswalk poles, street signs, and the brick sides of buildings, cutting Alyssa off constantly. Zero balance, agility, or grace. I am one of those vintage action figures made of segmented wooden squares and elastic string like nerves, but broken, wooden blocks not quite aligned, string twisted, cords rolling over notches of bone. Things pop, grind, lock, and slide. The old me was no gymnast, but I could at least stand and walk in a straight line.

My brain has forgotten how to compartmentalize stimuli. That genie is out of the bottle. The Ghost of April 7 orders me to look at everything all the time, especially the periphery. Checking and tracking. Checking for scary, terrible men reporting to an even scarier, more terrible man who wants to torture me out of a rightful settlement.

We pass a hipster craft beer bar yoga studio, a dive bar taco place, cigarette and wing joints, a dessert and quiche patisserie, high school team sport stores, antique galleries, a community theater, music shops with violin rental and guitar repair, some jewelers, a courthouse, and a

Catholic church. All drab, moss covered, quasi-European. I am not the only one with a limp, I notice. We are part of the pedestrian flow, flashing lights embedded in the road.

In every store window, next to chipping Open and Sales signs, I see my reflection. *That can't be me*, I think. But it is.

At the coffee shop, the handwritten chalkboard menu is enormous, so I just order a latte for the calcium. Alyssa gets an Americana. Out back is a little garden, a secluded coffee cove with graffitied walls—for paying patrons only, ever since it became the cute spot for freeloading senior pictures or save-the-dates. What looks to be an indie rock band is at one table, variations of black, tattered clothing, bandannas, pops of color in their rings, earrings, and nose piercings. They noticeably pause, evaluating us before resuming their conversation. Apparently, they know people who are performing across the street tonight at 7:00 p.m.

It's colder without direct sunlight, enclosed completely by the backs of buildings, but there's a bit of fairy-tale enchantment here. I like the fixed boundaries. I can keep track of everything. An old canoe is propped up in one corner, perhaps as an artistic or aesthetic statement. A stone cherub, arms folded under his young chin, looks up at me with a smile from the dirt and weeds.

"This is nice," I say, holding the paper cup with both hands, enjoying the texture of the cardboard sleeve. "It has been a while."

We sit. Talk about school for a minute. Eavesdrop.

"This shit happened like, a couple days ago, dude," one of the band members says to his table. "It wasn't on the news."

Alyssa and I exchange a wordless glance over our sips of coffee. Our non-verbal for *let's see where this goes.*

"I'm not sure if she was still pregnant or already had the kid. I think she already had it but whatever. Guy breaks a window, fucks up her husband, stabs him in the chest. Then into the baby's room," he continues.

I try to remain calm. Blink, stretch my eyelids. Trace the logo on the paper cup with my thumb.

"Slits mom's throat, fucking gush of blood. Sprays over all the walls.

Mutilates her body. Entrails, intestines all over the place, spilling the fuck out," he says, laughing.

I don't know what's happening. My hands are clammy. I can't sit still, pivoting and readjusting myself in the steel wire chair. Trying to crack my back in the same spot repeatedly.

I am me. I am her. I am the baby. I am the father, listening. I am back in time. Their blood is my blood too. I'm in the bedroom. Numb, blindsided, tackled into a pool of cough syrup. Logged with thick liquid while wearing layers of yarn. My ears buzz as if someone hit the monkey bars with a tree branch in my brain. I see myself getting stabbed where I got shot. Then cut into bits. I feel my scab tighten and burn. The sensation becomes chronic, caustic. My heart is dynamite in a coal mine, trying to excavate itself out.

"Her stomach looked like spaghetti. Still alive though—she's screaming, telling the guy not to hurt her baby. He did anyway. This dude murdered the whole family."

Alyssa's eyes ask, *Do you want to get out of here?*

Mine respond, *Yes.*

"Sorry about that," Alyssa says when we're gone. "Where to now? Want me to just bring you home?"

"Let's go to the pet store," I say.

We look at kittens, fish, hamsters, birds, and lizards. Seeing natural things, like outside, or animals, speeds up the recovery process, my surgeon says.

PAINFUL GAME

At times, my personal injury litigation feels like quarantine. Like house arrest. At other times, it feels like a full-time job. At all times, it is a terror-inducing deadlock, my entire life on hold. I've nicknamed this grueling part of my legal dilemma the Painful Game. In short, the Painful Game is the cold-blooded song and dance performed by insurance companies on a mission to settle for as little as possible, reeking of scare tactics, strategic delays, and medical artifice. Let me introduce you to its key members. There is a circuit of B-list (generous) doctors who are regularly hired by insurance companies to give biased reports on personal injury cases. They use strip mall clinics as a front with names like INTEGRITY MEDICAL EXAMS. To them, I am an invoice. To their masters, the insurance overlords, I am a claim number, a profit margin, a dollar amount that they will do everything in their power to mitigate, postpone, refute, or deny. This business is expressly dehumanizing. Were they to acknowledge the person, the life behind the paper and the numbers, they would not sleep at night.

Some exams take ten minutes, some take nine hours. Regardless, I convulse from anxiety each sleepless night before. Every waiting room is a panic attack. My lawyer has warned me that these doctors will be—are paid to be—skeptical of my symptoms. They may express doubt that I am injured or disabled at all. He says they may try to prove me wrong, and this thought is far worse than the examinations themselves.

The first thing I notice about these strip mall clinics is that they're mostly empty. No supplies, no medical paraphernalia, no cotton swabs or tongue depressors in readily available dispensers. The fact of the matter is they don't treat patients here. To the contrary, you sign a form agreeing to not be treated.

I hand this signed form and clipboard to the person at the front-desk, a woman in her eighties wearing a super-fuzzy pink turtleneck and one of those charm bracelets where each charm represents one of her grandchildren. I spot a baseball, a flower, and a cupcake. She has a lot of grandchildren.

The "doctor" is late, walks in disheveled from the snow, kicking off slush. He doesn't acknowledge me even though I'm the only person in the waiting room. This "doctor" doesn't even work here in any capacity. He's been brought in on a mercenary-like basis to give me the scammy once-over and isn't hiding it. From the moment I'm called into the exam room, I decide I will never call him doctor.

Just as I suspected, he brought all his own equipment: that goofy rubber reflex hammer, stethoscope, blood pressure monitor. These items are laid out meticulously on a desk. It's all for show.

"I'm not here to treat you, or help you in any way; you know that, right?" he says.

"Yes, I do," I say.

"Okay. With that out of the way, tell me what happened . . ." He trails off to check his notes. ". . . on the evening of April the 7, 2017."

"I got shot in the head," I say. My lawyer told me not to say anything beyond that. He said that the insurance company knows everything they need to know, and that any additional information I give them will be used against me.

"Surely there is more to it than that?" he says.

"Not that I know of," I say.

"I see," he says, writing way more than the words "got shot in head" on his notepad. "Let me get a look at you then."

He selects a tool that looks like a fat marker with a sharp but inkless point. He jabs it with force, first on my face, then hands, then feet.

"Can you feel that?" he asks.

My expression screams: *What do you think?*

He directs me to stick my elbows out as if gearing up to do the chicken dance, then pulls my arms back down to my sides.

"Don't let me move your arms," he says.

He gets aggravated when they come down easily.

"Try," he says.

"I am," I say, raising my eyebrows.

He tells me to take off my shoes and walk heel-toe across the examination room floor. On my way back, he tells me to do it with my eyes closed. I stumble, a real close call, and stick my arm out to brace for impact.

"Try," he says again, much more aggressively.

"I don't want to fall!"

Next, I must track his pen without moving my head. At this point, he is no different from a cop administering rudimentary DUI tests.

When it's over, I realize I shouldn't have worn these boots. The laces require multiple windings and knots around little nickel hooks, like a series of three miniature boat docks running parallel up the tongue of each foot. Like a clumsy pirate, I try to fasten everything down.

"Those boots look pretty sturdy," the "doctor" says as he makes a note on his clipboard. I assume he wrote something belittling.

All told, the exam took ten minutes. The "doctor" never once looked at my scans or read my medical history in full, although he no doubt earned a nice commission by delivering to Mark's insurance company a full-blown lengthy report deducing and extrapolating and classifying my injury as a mild TBI, nothing more.

PUBLIC SAFETY

For settlement purposes and perhaps a scrap of closure, too, I collect reports. The police report is easily obtained: I receive my own one-hundred-twenty-page copy, with pictures. But the University doesn't make anything easy. To my formal request, I am informed the University cannot release Public Safety reports off campus premises; they can only be reviewed under supervision. They will not mail it to my home address or send a digital file via email. They ask multiple times if, when I arrange a visit, anyone will accompany me, be it a third party or legal professional. They need to adhere to federal privacy laws and redact information from the report accordingly.

I think, *Well, fuck. You are actually making me come back again.*

—

Again, Mom and I don't want to pay the school three dollars for underground parking in the garage that once housed the gun that shot me, so we waste ten minutes cruising for a free spot on the street. This time, Mark's car is not in any nearby driveways. I pray he's moved back in with his parents, hours away from here.

I can't help but wonder about my room. There is no way the

University decommissioned the whole apartment, even if that would've been the thoughtful thing to do. I am sure they power-washed the blood, spackled and painted the walls. Some sophomore, in the dark about what happened, won't suspect a thing. That lucky sophomore will one day sit just beneath the still-hollow wall in the living room. He will bang his head against it after a long day of studying or miss a pass from his quarterback roommate, and the clay wood filler will come loose. It will pop out like a cork on a bottle of champagne. He will explore, looking for a hidden note, a message left just for him, maybe a long-lost fraternity secret. But it will be empty. And he will be disappointed. Until his roommate takes a pencil and draws some lines around the hole, deftly doodling a spread anus. And then, finally, they will laugh, taking turns pretending to finger it with their pinkies. Because that is what Mark and I would've done.

Mom and I take the elevator up to the third floor of a building that looks vaguely like a life-size jewelry display case: the Public Safety Department of the Dean of Students Office. A student is working the reception desk. I am dressed in the works. Knit hat, sunglasses, sour expression. Maneuvering with zero agility, speed, or grace. There isn't much progress in my physical recovery yet. Mom positions herself behind me in case I fall.

"I'm here to read a Public Safety report," I say, a little too defiantly. Mom and I are on the front lines here. If I am the Civil War horn blower, she is my drummer boy.

"Paul?" the student asks.

"You bet," I say, stuttering.

Emerging from an office, like a bear waking from hibernation, the man I have been in contact with via email. He is massive, an ex-football player or wrestler, maybe an alumnus. The impression he makes is of a man accustomed to being rewarded for violence and strength. I can tell he has never dealt with something this serious before. I am afraid to shake his hand. To maintain the illusion of confidence, I don't take my glasses off. We are both nervous and expectant.

"Hi, Paul. You can come right this way. I have the report ready for your review. I take it this is Mom?" he says.

"Kathi," Mom introduces herself, shakes his hand.

We sit down in what amounts to a police interrogation room. There are no windows. Everything is gray and plastic with that ubiquitous weird wispy design that looks like someone ruffled a fuzzy black blanket over every surface.

"So," he begins, "got any plans for the summer? Vacations anywhere?"

It has been two months to the day since I was shot in the head.

"No," I say. "I can't really do anything."

"No," Mom says with a glare. "We are staying home."

"Well, let me get that report all laid out," he says, awkward as ever. He looks at Mom. "Kathi, you said you are not reading any documents today, correct?"

"Correct. I brought my own book to read."

I set a pencil and notebook beside me. I'm fairly sure note-taking is not allowed. I didn't plan on it, but it's my small, mighty protest.

"Okay. So, here's everything. Take as much time as you need."

———

There are three separate packets, write-ups and information from various interviews and officer accounts. As I crease over the first page, I can't believe all this is about me.

It reads like an old fable; it's just missing a moral. Go ahead and lie, you can get away with it. I skip over the Public Safety officer's name. I don't want to hate her.

As I read what Mark said in his interviews, I find my body mirroring his actions, his mannerisms. My hands are shaking. I am sweating, nauseated. I feel faint, fuzzy, and gray, like the pattern in the furniture. The room is dead silent. The man is watching me closely. I can feel him staring at the top of my head, checking out my crater and scar. Mom has her book open to a random page but is watching me and crying.

I page through everything. Some of it overlaps with the police reports. After forty-five minutes, I call it quits. Legally, nothing amounts from this. But here it is what factually happened, on paper and ink. Do with it what you will.

The man gives me a smile that I interpret as: *I realize this might not be the last time we hear from you.*

I think: *I never want to see you or this place ever again.*

In the main lounge, I pull out my notebook. Mom is on lookout, checking to see if the man is still watching us from the third-floor balcony.

While I write in a little frenzy, Mom asks if there was anything new.

This is what it says, verbatim, publicly accessed from the document I had just read, now on the University's Public Safety crime report website and available online.

04/07/2017 at 6:48–6:57. Public Safety responded to a localized fire alarm in [redacted] Residence Hall. A [University] student claimed to have used an electronic vaporizer in the residence in violation of University Policy.

04/07/2017 at 6:46–11:00. Public Safety, [the police], [the fire department], and medics responded to a medical in [redacted] Residence Hall. A [University] student who was injured by the negligent discharge of a firearm was transported by medics to an area hospital for further medical care.

So.

At 6:46, they respond to a "medical," which they determine is an injury due to the negligent discharge of a firearm.

At 6:48, a Public Safety officer responds to the fire alarm in my residence hall, which she determines is due to an electronic vaporizer.

At 8:45ish, Mark (finally) calls for help.

These three things cannot all be true.

8:45 is true, supported by Mark and witnessed by Keith, Rachel, the Public Safety officer who went on her merry way, the first responders who took me to the hospital, and the medical professionals who admitted me to emergency care.

6:46 cannot be true. Yet, that is the time they claim the "medical" began.

"So they lied. Make note of that," Mom says. "Anything else?"

I break the hours down for her: what Mark did while I was blacked out, his string of lies to Public Safety, this path to 8:45ish, the time he wasted before getting help.

Mom starts to cry. She makes a fist. Her eyes are fierce.

"I want to beat his fucking ass," she says.

I get choked up. I don't think I've ever seen Mom in such a state of feral, protective aggression. As disappointed as I am with Mark, pissed off by the obvious, I'm more upset that his past choices have made Mom feel so sad, so angry, so sorry for me. I'm glad she's in my corner, but at the same time, I feel a sense of guilt about her acting this way on my behalf. Though maybe Mark deserves it. My mom's tough. She's from Detroit. If they ever did run into each other on the street, my bets would be on her.

FRIENDSHIP III

"First things first. Are you hungry? Let's get snacks."

We swiped our student IDs, filled with what felt like free money even though it was part of our tuition. Our usual haul: chocolate bars embedded with dried raspberries, Sanpellegrino Limonata, and extra-tender beef jerky filets. With student loans, I'm still paying for those snacks right now.

We hopped into a Ping-Pong tournament. Played some billiards. Mark, Keith, and I were finally able to catch up. Mark had gone overseas to study abroad. Keith had stayed on campus for a public speaking course. I opted out of J-term and spent the month of January working at an upholstery shop owned by my brother-in-law, stripping furniture from hospital waiting rooms and corporate offices. I was bunking at Krystin's house, roiling in my anxiety over handling razor blades, afraid of losing a finger.

Mark went first. That year, it was an entrepreneurship course in India; the year prior, business management in the UK. I never studied abroad because I couldn't afford it, a fact they both knew, though it was never openly discussed. Mark showed how the new tattoo he got on his shoulder was made up of a bunch of individual dots and told us how the bartenders nicknamed him Fireball by the third day, for obvious reasons. He was proud. I wasn't a huge fan of how proud.

Chatting about travel goals, Mark's country of birth came up. He knew nothing about his parents other than that they had been living overseas for a time. He said yes, that country would be cool to visit. But he had no interest in locating his biological parents. They separated their lives from me for a reason, he said. And for once, he was quiet. Then he made an obnoxious groan like two wild boars making love over hot coals. A subversion. The Do Not Enter sign pasted on the bulkhead door to his raw, unfiltered emotions.

Mark believed he was vulnerable when he wasn't joking around, which was in my estimation not quite accurate, but he preferred to be strong, performative, pursuing his hijinks without emotional commitment to anyone or anything. I did not then and will not now pretend to understand the hardships he endured, the hardships that come with being adopted, the racism he no doubt has dealt with his entire life. I wish I could have been more of an ally, as well as a best friend.

Something I've come to find out quite recently, it really does help to talk about it.

The problem is, Mark took it out on others, just as I have in the wake of the shooting. During our run together my skin got thick. The constant roughhousing ceased to hurt. The never-really-listening, the glib juvenile responses, each one a variation of *I'm naked underneath my clothes*, ceased to annoy. The names he called me—fucking slut, dickhole, piece of shit—I knew he was kidding, he was always kidding, but hearing it that many times a day, every day, wore on me until they, too, ceased to hurt. The jokes he made about my dad kicking me out as a kid ceased to hurt. I became so tempered I could stop bullets. At some point, my head might stop hurting too.

There was hesitation at first, sure. But at the time, I wrote it off as Mark acting like the curmudgeonly grandpa, or the boy who picks on you in grade school, only giving you a hard time because deep down, he has a crush on you. He would insult me like a sailor then reach out for what felt like an honest, heartfelt hug. I'm sure that affected my psyche, crossed some wires in an unhealthy way. I'd only ever had one other best friend before, so I figured this was just how things were now, the modern way to josh around. I regret ignoring the litany of red flags presented to me.

He loved making a scene. "*Sun's out, guns out!*" he'd yell to some football players walking toward the gym, all pecs and arms. "*Hey, Dad!*" in the face of a girl trying to have a quiet phone conversation on her walk to wherever. Keith and I would snicker from behind, both of us along for the ride. "I bet she can't *stand* that," he'd say in front of a girl in a motorized wheelchair. Always judging, always in the guise of a prank.

I, like any aspiring writer, simply observed.

Mark was a living, breathing comments section in need of constant stimulation. He was an American Troll. For a good while, he flooded that behavior into my life. He normalized it. Keith and I became quick on our toes, quick with a venomous joke, to keep up; everyone was fat, stupid, ugly, or boring. Sometimes all four at once.

On some level, I knew it was wrong, that these things were cruel. I'd think, *This wasn't me three years ago.* But I was far too submerged in him and invested in our relationship to confront the change. He was my roommate. The first person to approach me in college and actively want to become friends. These things felt set in stone. I couldn't imagine starting over with someone else.

We played video games, friendly fire always on. World wars, zombies, stealth action, nuclear fallout. When a game wasn't multiplayer, Keith and I would bring our PlayStations to the living room where Mark's Xbox was. We routed them to some computer monitors on the coffee table, and set up camp right there, ducks in a row, just so we could play independently and together at the same time.

On the couch, Mark deposited spit into a Mellow Yellow bottle, suds tainted brown from pouches of dipping tobacco. Keith and I both hounded him to quit chewing. He'd say haphazardly, "I know; I just really want mouth cancer." You could smell the tobacco-mint mixed with hot breath right before he'd screw on the cap and wedge the bottle in the cushion between us.

One night, while virtually hunting terrorists, the three of us came up with the plot of a short story, about a drug-dealing hamster who lives in a teenager's shirt pocket. The hamster was so obviously the one in charge, barking commands at the teen, who was playing hooky at a space-themed arcade. Chaos ensues. Things do not go as planned. If I remember correctly, the hamster dies by freak accident. Gets run over by a car.

I wrote the story. Neither Keith nor Mark ever read it. They had no interest in my writing. Maybe they were afraid it would be bad, knowing how much I banked on becoming a writer. Either way, the plot made them laugh. And Mark's laugh was something I've never heard anywhere else. It had no distinct syllables like *ha ha*; just air. A gust shot out though the nostrils like an empty whipped cream aerosol canister, still with a bit of CO_2 locked inside. The air Mark pushed out seemed to inflate his eyes. With every laugh, another pump.

Mark had a benign tumor surgically removed some years ago, tucked way up in his nasal cavity. The same nasal cavity his laugh came from. Perhaps it's all related.

Every so often he left school to go to a special hospital miles away for tests and scans. Making sure it didn't grow back. When he returned with good news, the three of us celebrated by noodling some blues jams and getting seven-layer burritos. He'd ask if I smelled what he was smelling, some foul odor, a bizarre aftereffect of the procedure again. A mix of balsamic vinegar and ground-up SweeTARTS. Nine out of ten times he asked, it was just his nose.

I hope he's healthy. I hope he quit chewing for good. And for God's sake, I hope he stopped making all those dumb jokes.

FORGETFULNESS

One night, a couple months post-injury, everyone was over for dinner and complaining. I was on the couch with a blanket over my face, watching my family converse through a gap in the stitching.

Krystin said she was tired, didn't want to work anymore, wanted to get paid to watch her kids at home.

Anna agreed, not about watching the kids, but about the not-working thing. She talked about sitting too long and how that contributes to her less-than-ideal posture. "There is, like, this really weird thing that happens with my lower back. The lower left corner, above my hip. I know I sit wrong. And then I get a headache."

"I've been getting headaches a lot lately too!" Alyssa said. "I got a really bad one at Rebecca's baby shower." Which then reminded her of something. "Paul, why were you acting so weird when I brought Rebecca over here the other day? You didn't even say hi."

I know it is not fair to make headaches off-limits. I do not reign supreme over things that hurt. I know I'm not the grand pillar of suffering. All bad things do not need to be measured by my personal standard of bad. I try not to clear my throat every time someone mentions *head* and *pain* in the same sentence. Pointing out that I was acting strange lately was a cheap shot though. Because of *course* I was. A bullet had struck my skull. I'm still a little sensitive about that.

The blanket slunk down to my stomach as I sat up. I became Hulkish, eyes narrowing, hands making fists. I wanted to lash out but the most I could physically muster was to maybe throw a pillow across the room. Again, there exists this paradox between how I appear and how I am. Look at me: staples removed, hair growing back, scar slowly receding beneath. My appetite has returned. I'm filling out. Walking more than seven steps at a time. I don't need sunglasses indoors anymore. When I'm with my niece, asking about preschool, less often do I need to plug my ears to temper the noise and stimulation of an energetic child who doesn't always remember to use a soft voice around Uncle Paul.

That superpower wore off too. That survival bounce—that feeling that I could do anything—that miracle aura of *you'll never believe what happened to me*. It was fading.

Time marched on, but I never de-escalated. I was perpetually experiencing the shooting 24/7. Any measurable progress was an illusion. I was simply getting used to the new normal. I held on to this pettiness for a long while after what happened. Indulging is preferable to the pain of trauma. To be dismissive, angry, resentful, felt perversely powerful. The superiority of the brain injured. Your back hurts from sitting too long in an office chair? Toothache? Migraine? You attention seeker. Fuck you. You know nothing of misery.

Around that time, whatever long-distance complaining event I thought I was running, it turns out life is a relay race. I had no choice but to pass the complaining baton to Mom. Her brother, my Uncle Ray, died of cancer that started in his hip and spread to his lungs. Her sister, my Aunt Claire, had an inoperable brain aneurysm that could burst and kill her instantly, and she was scrambling for second opinions. Mom's ninety-four-year-old mother, fifteen hours away by car, was barely getting by; any money Mom sent, well, her other brother took some of it for cigarettes.

Eight hours away by car in the opposite direction, my dad was taking Mom to court in an attempt to end his spousal-support duties.

Don't forget the thing about her son that had just happened, which I was trying to remember was *not* the sum of everything terrible in the entire world.

"Maybe I should just take work off and go home for a while," Mom said. She was working through all this. Home meaning Detroit, where her family still lived. "But I can't, realistically, because your father would track me down, send me hate mail. And I need money for a lawyer. And I can't take any more time off work, I'm worried they'll fire me if I keep asking."

With that, she made a finger gun with her thumb and pointer, placed the barrel above her ear, and gave imaginary weight to the noiseless trigger pull. She jolted her head to dramatize the recoil and aftershock, the space for blood spatter.

"Just shoot me," she said.

My vision zoomed out, a fish-eye lens over my head. This bowed, expanding sensation moved to my stomach, followed by a tingle that might be like drinking a glass full of steel wool shavings. I looked for the nearest mirror. Checked for the hole, found a scab-covered crater now. The dead giveaways went away, but the daily reminders did not. If fact, they became more diverse; they multiplied.

"I'm so sorry," Mom said, realizing her mistake. Her shoulders slouched forward, head draped to one side, eyes closed in a full-body wince. "Damnit."

Everyone's face soured. I was momentarily satisfied by their pity until we all felt miserable again.

EXPELLED II

My lawyer sent me an email. He said Mark graduated after being expelled. The University allowed him to come back in the summer and finish school. Mark graduated and has his degree. We have diplomas from the same institution. They let *him* back on campus; they wouldn't help *me*, the victim, but they'll help Mark, the wrongdoer. They let him come back and rewarded him.

I didn't get much in terms of details, but it's not hard to speculate. Possibly, Mark appealed the expulsion and won. He has money. He could have hired a lawyer to contest the University's decision. That happens all the time. But this lack of respect, this change of heart, almost feels targeted. I feel like I'm being made the fool—both by Mark's audacity to attempt a comeback with options galore and the school's flimsy backbone to maintain conviction. A double whammy, this one stings extra.

Though I will never change my mind about pressing charges, the properties that make up my hurt have changed on the premise of intention. This is not the course of action of someone who promised to help me. I no longer believe that Mark is acting with my best interests in mind. And as we get deeper and deeper into the trenches of personal injury law, that realization feels a lot like a threat.

DATE

My first date since the shooting: I'm going out to eat with Anna, god-damnit, if it's the last thing we do. Which it very well might be.

Overcome with paranoia, it took me forever to leave the house. I thought we were being followed the entire way here.

I ask Anna if she thinks I lost my twinkle.

She says maybe. She says my face for sure looks sadder. Maybe I'm more critical now too? Down-to-earth? Realistic? I don't fool around anymore, is how we diagnose it. Hypervigilant, suspicious, too cynical to play games. I always feel like I'm doing something wrong, something illegal, just by living. For me, quiet-sad is now very on-brand, replacing anti-Trump skits and testicle jokes, which is a major change.

My hair is creeping up past completely sheared. I am entrusting Krystin to cut and shape it as it continues to grow. She considers herself an amateur stylist. I can sort of fluff the front upward a bit with sculpting paste to make it resemble a small, homemade skate-board ramp.

A hostess asks us how many are in our party and I feel a hefty Spiral coming on. I've noticed similar feelings when helping Mom shop for groceries. Things churn, and accumulate, often in public.

The phases of a typical Spiral:

1) Due to Traumatic Brain Injury, overstimulation creates deep and precise physical pain.

2) Due to Painful Game, paranoia is generated by any and all life that might be enjoyed, particularly life lived out of doors, and I must pay obsessive attention to detail, Checking and Tracking everything and everyone around me.

3) Due to Checking and Tracking, I am returned to phase 1, which now runs hog wild.

Spiral.

We are seated.

Within the Spiral, a bone headache hits, a Mini-Spiral, a Sub-Spiral. I will get uptight, take it out on others, which is to say, Anna.

I rub a newly discovered plateau near the peak of my forehead with my first and middle finger. My head is two warring plate tectonics doing battle over my scar. Angry, empty neurons fire to nowhere. My own inverted Battle of the Bulge, in miniature. I want to peel off my skin and smooth out a truce.

I don't want to be here. I can tell Anna does, but not like this.

Our waiter comes and I ask if he can point me in the direction of the restroom. He plays around that they got rid of it last night; I'm a day late and a dollar short.

I don't sympathy laugh. I don't smile or joke back. I don't say, *Guess I'll have to shit in the freezer!* I just wait. He's just having fun! No. I've had real fun, with Mark, laughing until we piss ourselves, from the stupidest stuff. This is artificial fun with a stranger who is trying too hard. This is a waste of time. This is wrong.

After fifteen seconds he points that way, now aware I don't play games anymore.

I collect water from the faucet in my hand and drip some down the back of my neck.

A few minutes pass and I return. Anna gives me her tucked-lip smile like a folded blanket. The kind she does when she's trying to be polite but knows something's off. I think she's fed up with me. I wish she were more perceptive. She wishes I wasn't angry about everything. I take offense but know it's my fault. It can be deceiving. My body is getting better, but my mind is getting worse. As things heal and reconnect, the more brain-power there is to fuel my trauma. The more it manipulates me.

Her eyes say: *I'll try not to treat you any differently now*, which I both admire and disdain at the same time.

My eyes say: *Pick something to eat already.*

We finger through the menu. I twitch every time the restaurant door opens. Jump back, startled, whenever someone scooches out their chair. Every face is the face of somebody following me. There is too much sound and activity. I wish everyone in the restaurant would just agree to take turns taking bites.

"Are we celebrating anything today?" the waiter asks once we are ready to order.

"Nothing in particular," Anna and I both say.

No promotions. No marriage proposals. No birthdays. No pretend birthdays for a free dessert. Not the wonder and beauty of life itself nor the appreciation of said beauty. No games.

I wait for a water refill, ripping at my cuticles like little bits of dried glue. No alcohol anymore. Ever. The thought of getting buzzed does nothing for me, to be honest.

Anna orders a gin gimlet and flatbread pizza. I order fish since I read online that omega-3 fatty acids are good for a traumatic brain injury.

The waiter leaves after writing down our entrées. Anna looks at me. I look at her silverware.

Both our eyes say: *Well, at least we're here.*

THERAPY II

For a week I thought it was heart related.

I'd be sitting on the couch, phone against my thigh, and I'd look down at a just-checking-in text from Anna. Then it would strike.

A surge of some kind. The world's smallest lightning bolt. Followed by five seconds of numbness. Starting in the shoulder, then down into my fingertips. On the left side. That's heart related, right? I'm going to have a heart attack. I hastily draft a bucket list before asking Krystin what it could be if not impending doom. She says it's probably not heart related. Probably something to do with my nerves. She urges me to go to the doctor.

My primary care guy, who has already prescribed me a selective serotonin reuptake inhibitor for anxiety and major depressive disorder, says he might have an idea and shows me a stretch where he juts his chin out and then tucks it in at the top of his chest. He looks like a giant, self-loading PEZ Dispenser. I try it and get a few pops and cracks.

Primary Care Guy says it may be a bulged vertebra, resulting from crashing into a well-made dining room chair after the bullet's impact. My image of a Pez Dispenser is reinforced. He says if the zap and numbness don't go away in one week, come back and he'll do some X-rays.

I go back for some X-rays. He aligns my neck and spine. Yes, I have a bulged disk. And maybe something more. He gives me a referral for physical therapy.

Jen, the physical therapist, has read my records in full and she treats everything matter-of-factly, saying things like, *You must have been so scared, your mom must have been worried sick*, etcetera, all calm and cool and somewhat devoid of emotion.

Jen asks me some questions.

Symptoms? Look down, zap and numbness. Tiny lightning bolt. Thought it might be heart related. Happy it's not. I almost delegated my belongings.

Any other symptoms? Yes. I have plenty, but the zap is why I'm here. I don't want Jen to bite off more than she can chew. I'm entrusting her with a big task as is. But for whatever reason, she insists on hearing the rest.

Well, headaches, for one. All different kinds. Front, side, between the eyes. Plate tectonic tissue and bone ones, you name it. Poor sleep. Mental fatigue, exhaustion. Physical inability to do daily tasks. A stupid number of psychological issues. I drop things randomly and run into walls a lot.

She has ambitious plans to tackle everything. But first things first. A general examination with instruments that look straight out of an eighth-grade geometry classroom.

Jen measures my movements with a protractor and rearranges my limbs to test potential diagnoses. During this procedure, we break the ice.

She asks what I do. I say I'm a writer. She is taken by surprise. She is glad. She says I'll be able to describe what I'm feeling better than most because I write.

I fuss with my crater. Jen asks if I touch it often. I say it's compulsive. A built-in, inverted stress ball. Out of nowhere she says she has a daughter in college. That's nice, I say, unsure if she is trying to set us up.

Jen tells me to lift my head a certain way and hold my left arm up. I feel a mega zap, a short tingle, then it goes numb for five seconds. I relay this information.

"You have thoracic outlet syndrome. The bone and muscle around your neck in this area are cutting off blood circulation, as well as a bundle of nerves, sending a zap and tingling sensation to your left arm, hand, and fingers. It comes from the muscle tension that often accompanies the gesture to protect one's head."

"That makes a lot of sense," I say. It appears I've been protecting my head, chronically so.

There is a surgery she can recommend where they remove a chunk of the collarbone. I choose a couple months of stretching.

Once a week, Jen mirrors me to help make the moves less awkward. We do median nerve and ulnar nerve and scalene muscle stretches. Some yoga—seated cat cow and child's pose. We wall crawl. We do sit-stands with my arms crossed over my chest for limited space cardio. We put the palms of our hands together, as if praying with a rosary, and move that side to side across our torsos. We place a finger in a particular spot on our lower necks to hold down a tendon, and turn, looking upward, to stretch it. My nerves are piano strings and my fingers the keys. I stretch till it sings.

We do doorway pectoral major and doorway pectoral minor stretches where it looks like I'm very indecisive about entering the room. Jen says my arms are weak, a subscriber to the maxim that one must first have muscles before you can stretch them. We do band workouts, out in the hallway, using her closed door to hold the bands in place. I don't understand why we can't switch which side the bands are on, so I don't have to be out in the hall, but this is how she sets it up, every time. Other patients speed walk behind as I pump away, three sets of rows and erected pulls.

Jen wants to address my dizziness and fatigue and eyestrain by having me track a moving pen for sixty seconds. We use my ability to watch Timberwolves games as a gauge of progress.

"I had to look away a lot, but I could watch the whole thing this time," I say.

"That's great," she says, completely deadpan.

It's tough to pin down what Jen really thinks of me. I know she cares that I got shot, but I sense hints of sarcasm in her cool, calm, and collected voice.

She leads me to a room littered with perfectly aligned, crisp Post-it notes all over the walls, as if it were the apartment of a tidy conspiracy theorist. There is a small foam square in the middle of the floor.

"This is a laser pointer," she says, showing me the laser pointer in her palm. "This is how I am going to indicate which Post-it you need to focus on. You are to focus on that note, while balancing one-footed on that foam square, for five seconds. Then, I will indicate another note, and so on."

As I take my place on the square, I'm nervous that this will make me an even more elite Checker and Tracker of settlement agents. On the upside, it will help me watch basketball games without experiencing any pain. I don't know if this is a wash, but I do what she says.

To improve my sleep, she recommends a memory foam contour pillow. To manage my headaches, manual desensitization therapy. She grabs a lock of my hair and tugs on it while making concentric circles. She says this will give my head new and harmless sensations to relearn. She massages my scar tissue and crater and says I should do the same with various household objects. I picture myself rubbing a TV remote all over my head and face and giggle.

While she's using two hands and all her body weight to push on my spine, I tell her about the Timberwolves' recent five-game win streak in staggered, breathy grunts. Jen says she can tell by how flexible my spine is that I don't smoke. It goes on like this for twelve weeks.

Jen asks me at the end of each session if I've improved since I first came in. I say yes, the rest of my body really is starting to feel better. Other than headaches, my only real hang-ups are daily screen-fatigue and overstimulation that I usually try to walk off.

She asks about PTSD. I tell her, unfortunately, as my body has gotten better my mind has gotten worse. But she's done a lot, and I'm thankful. I move my arm like I just got a new one sewed on, testing out rotations. I feel around where the imaginary stitching would be.

"I go to talk therapy," I say. "Often on the same days I see you." It's all a part of Paul's Comprehensive Recovery Plan. "We are trying to figure that stuff out."

I tell her I'm thinking about applying to grad school, try and fail to explain how the fully funded ones work, something I don't fully understand myself. They only take like six students, I say, and you sort of teach entry-level literature classes on the side. No, they pay you to do it. Like $18,000 a year. More if you help run their literary magazine. There is no tuition.

As cool as ever, she says, "It's nice to have dreams."

INTERVIEW

I drive thirty-five minutes to a drab three-story corporate building in a city I know only by name, located just outside of Minneapolis. I'm driving now, again. And not unlike the first time Mom taught me how to drive, she made me go through a mini driver's ed before giving me full approval.

I park, a little nervous for my interview, already missing the smell of the interior of my car, ready to cry like a newborn in the unadulterated light of day.

I am wearing a gray suit. The jacket is from Goodwill and Mom bought me the pants for Christmas last year, but thankfully the shades of gray are close enough in hue to pass as a matching set. My hair is short, could be considered normal for a business setting, but I'm no fan yet.

I clutch a leather-bound folder containing my resume. It belongs to Anna. It is a University folder. I'm banking on their reputation: strong business program, excellent hiring rate after graduation. I have mixed feelings every time I look at the insignia.

Honestly, I don't know much about the company. From their website, I gather they do emergency environmental construction work, and that they need an English major as a marketing and communications intern.

Kate, director of marketing and communications, and Nick, a graphic designer and the only other person on the marketing team, welcome me into a conference room.

Kate is friendly and does most of the talking, weaving in and out of standard corporate phrases. Nick is younger, calmer. They are the perfect team. One is a bolt of electricity. The other a sheath of rubber.

The chairs in this room are the same ones you see on TV, in board-room or important-pitch scenes. For the first time in my life, I feel like what I say matters.

Kate wants to get to know me a little. She asks about hobbies. She asks where I went to school.

I answer truthfully. Kate does not mention the shooting. Because Kate doesn't know it happened. Not too many people do.

"Even though you're an English major, you probably still know what ROI is, from osmosis of going there, right?"

"Absolutely."

I have no idea.

"Return on investment," Kate says after a long pause.

"Exactly," I say.

I am charming once I get going. A real schmoozer. Kate tells me the company is in serious need of proper messaging. No one thinks big picture. All the tech experts are too focused on repeat transactional commodity work. She says they are very granular, siloed, and entrepreneurial. She says they get in the weeds easily and marketing is the group that is supposed to stay thirty thousand feet above. She says they are going from four companies to one.

She says they need better copy, pronto. She says I'll need to make landfills seem sexy. She says I'll have to interview scientists and engineers, and extract a story out of things like, we dug a hole here and then filled it with concrete, then put a flag on it, and billed the client.

I say that all sounds fun, I'm excited for the opportunity. I mean it.

"What's the biggest challenge you've overcome?" Nick asks.

I don't want to tell them exactly, but I want to seal the deal.

"I recently had a serious injury, an accident, where I could have died, but here I am, talking to you guys. It has been a crazy couple of months, but I think I'm gradually becoming better because of it." I stutter a bit, one of my more noticeable residual symptoms, but the point gets across.

They are stunned, wowed. Kate says interns are capped off at thirty hours a week and make eighteen bucks an hour. I am stunned, wowed. I've never had more than five hundred dollars in my bank account.

They ask if I have any questions. I am bad at asking questions. Where do I sign?

Kate tells me I'll hear back if I'm selected no later than Wednesday, two days from now.

For the sole purpose of seeing her happy, I drive to Mom's office right after my interview and, hoping my gut feeling is right, tell her I got the job. I haven't seen her face this lively, this happy since before the shooting. She introduces me to her coworkers, gluing me close in a one-arm hug. All the people who were so kind with gift baskets and flowers and time off, meeting me now, in person, for the first time.

"He got the job!" Mom proudly proclaims. They congratulate me quietly, respectful that I'm still sensitive to overstimulation. Even their mannerisms are quiet, slow, and soft. A soft office nod, a tender hand-shake. Everyone seems to be keeping as still as possible.

"The interview went well," I say. "I was nervous in the car beforehand, but once I got talking it was all fine. The lady who would potentially be my boss said they need a writer to make landfills seem sexy." Mom laughs.

"I'm so proud of you, honey," Mom says.

Wednesday, at the latest.

BASKETBALL III

For a taste of the sacred act, for some beautiful uncontested thinking time where the body flows and the mind roams free, synced up as one by the rhythm of a bouncing sphere, I drive out to a park near my sister's house. I've dreamed for years about using this park as a setting for a story, something about a werewolf that lives in a dumpster and is caught in a time loop.

Though it would take more than a few sessions on the court to do so, I am determined to level up my strength, balance, agility. According to the regulars who flock my local community center who refuse to call me anything but Luka Dončić, I have. Step-back threes, reverse layups, turnaround jumpers, behind-the-back bounce passes—I've hit some nasty game winners and dropped some meaty dimes. Cautious regarding my head, I stay back in terms of defense.

The basketball court is tucked away in the woods, and I dodge tree branches to get there. It's like the court of an ogre or fun-loving cannibal, right next to their gingerbread house or cozy swamp. There's privacy. But I keep an eye out for people lurking between the trees. Checking and Tracking, one can never be too careful.

I decide to run killers. I want to see what my body can endure.

I start doing reps, inbounds line to inbounds line. After I work up a lather, I switch to left-handed layup drills, followed by lateral quickness shuffle runs in the paint. I try some novice ballhandling tricks and the ball bounces into a bush. Irate, I punt the ball over a fence, into the tennis courts.

Hands on my knees, panting, my limbs feel filled with those sun-baked playground pebbles near the slide. I'd never hobbled over to my duffle bag for a drink of water so fast.

I had never known tired. I had never known hot, or uncoordinated. I was meeting tiers of exhaustion that surpassed anything I'd ever experienced.

The cannibal witch next door just threw me out of her cauldron, needing meat not bones, knowing titanium spoils the soup.

Lost in my head, I don't notice him until he's under the chain net, a young physically disabled boy in a mobility scooter. Though we are merely ten feet away, he doesn't see me.

Thin wire glasses sit on the tip of his nose; he has boxy features, and an electric-green shirt that might be the result of searching for stock images tagged ROBOT BATTLE FUN.

We stay in silent proximity for a while. He seems to have come to admire the great outdoors, and like me, the quaint privacy this particular spot provides. I remain hunched, drained, replenishing breath as if I have just emerged from the bottom of the ocean, when he spots me in his peripheral vision. He's surprised. He puckers his lips and lowers them in tandem. A sort of alarmed frown.

I freeze, unsure what to do.

"Sorry," the boy says, as if entering the wrong classroom, and he turns to go.

I have the urge to shout, *Wait! What's up?* I don't want him to leave on my account. We could've chatted. I could've asked him if he had any interest in basketball, what his favorite team was, favorite player. I could've asked him if he wanted to chill and take a few shots, hang out for a bit. But we both refused to interrupt the other.

By many accounts, a near-death experience changes a person. Opens them up to life. Increases their compassion. It is also known that traumatic brain injury does just the opposite, decreasing emotional intelligence and empathy. I've been pulled by these opposing forces, not sure which team I play for. My life has been reduced to dualities. Life/death. Courage/fear. Forgiveness/hatred. Love/anger. Laugh/cry. I'm never sure if I'm supposed to wish April 7 never happened, or just adapt and be thankful. The answer is yes.

This was a perfect opportunity to prove to myself that I was not the same squirrely asshole anymore. A chance to prove that I was trying, that, alongside my physical skills, I was improving emotionally. Getting better at being inclusive, less passive, more open. A quick conversation could have gone a long way, any dignified response even. Instead, silence. I didn't even have the nerve to try.

Disabled in different ways, this boy didn't realize how much we had in common.

Through a break in the trees, I spy a black SUV pulling into the parking lot a good hundred yards away. I do not want to go home yet. Exercise, however taxing, is a godsend. But it's not up to me.

I've deduced that private investigators and settlement agents tend to buy American. Pretending to stretch, I creep a little closer. Toyota. This is not as bad as a Chrysler, Ford, Jeep, or the worst offender, Cadillac, but not nearly as good as a Volkswagen, Honda, Mazda, or Volvo. Only one shadowy figure in the car. Never good. Two people or better yet, a dog, I can relax. I can't relax. I can't see if they're in athletic gear or a dress shirt. The driver refuses to emerge. I make an executive decision to flee.

I walk past at a distance, shielding the ball behind my back, head down, doing my best to hide any distinguishing features on my body. I memorize the license plate and add it to my mental database of vehicles to avoid in the future. On the bright side: Minnesota plates. Not a sure sign but better than Wisconsin. Wisconsin, home to the headquarters of Mark's insurance company and its attendant torture chambers.

WORK

Kate calls me. I put it on speaker and hold the phone very far away from my head. She relays the following.

I'll be writing copy for services like Hydrocarbon Reclamation and Feasibility Analyses using words like *municipality*, *infrastructure*, and *custom tailored, comprehensive solutions*. Just like my creative, everyday writing, I'll have to try and make these words sound good together, with a business casual, consistent voice. I hear people go nuts for alliteration.

I'll be tasked with interviewing scientists and engineers to write project profiles for eighteen-million-dollar canola-oil facilities. Populate the website and post to social.

I'll be fairly compensated for my skill set.

I'll be the firm's youngest employee.

I'll be sharing a cube with Nick—the building is a little low on space right now, but I'll get my own laptop, extra monitor, wired keyboard, wired mouse, wired phone, branded coaster, branded coffee mug, branded water bottle, branded whiskey glass, branded can koozie, branded pizza cutter, branded water-wicking golf towel, branded T-shirt, branded polo, and branded zip-up that is also water-wicking. I get health insurance, and a beloved 401(k).

Marketing, now consisting of Kate, Nick, and me, will go out for a team-building lunch on the company credit card the last Friday of every month, somewhere nice, with vegan options for Kate.

I'll be working a maximum of thirty hours a week, with Tuesdays off for my therapy and doctor appointments. She understands. Breaks are encouraged every hour. Walk up and down the stairs, get a sip of water, get away from the screens, whatever I need when my head starts to hurt, if my eyes feel like they're being inflated with a bike pump. Any mental exhaustion or dizziness. Care, paired with a total lack of curiosity, is new, thrilling. My colleagues will have no "before" to compare to this me that is "after."

Surely nothing can go wrong.

MOVING OUT

Mom mentions now might be a good time to fly the coop. I'm surprised, and for a second, a little sad. But I have an email signature and a girl-friend. I'm stable and steadily improving, according to my doctors, and she doesn't need to be a nurse at my side any longer.

Anna and I pick a cheap place in a complex called Crystal Village, which we immediately begin to call Crystal Meth Village. When asked where we live, Anna and I will answer half-truthfully, saying we live on the border of the nicer suburban city next door.

It's not big, but it's not too small. New cabinets and paint. We're told the carpets have been shampooed. It has a sliding glass door that opens to a shallow deck hovering no more than a foot above a row of cars, with a picturesque view of the vast parking lot. No matter, our blinds will be eternally pulled shut—no settlement agents or private investigators will ever catch a glimpse of Paul's Special Wii Golf Time, where I do ten push-ups, twenty sit-ups, and fifty calf-raises between each hole. I just know these agents have their own depraved social media where they post pictures of the people they are being paid to watch, our silly damaged lives a scroll of amusement.

Sure, the pipes bang like they are going to burst. Yeah, the lack of central air-conditioning is kind of a drag. So what if the power goes out about once a week? Maybe a little more counter space would be nice, but this is being picky. Then there's Beverly. Our neighbor.

"I didn't know people could move in mid-month" is how she introduced herself.

"Oh, you know, they, um, prorate rent," I said, as we shook hands, awkward as I've ever been. Single, elderly, she blares her TV whenever she is home, at any hour. Through the wall, the constant cadence of newscasters sounds like they have wet rags in their mouths. (We place bets on what she does during the day, where she goes. I guess DJ at an underground elderly wrestling club. It would explain why she can't hear her TV. Anna thinks she is a palm reader.)

Beverly is not great for my TBI, but at least we have our own space. Anna's commute is fifteen minutes; I could walk to work if I had to. I'm almost self-sufficient and have Anna in case of emergency. And she has me, though mostly I piss her off eating Oreos, open-faced and manually double-stuffing; I then put the uneaten cookie halves back in the sleeve, too ashamed to throw them in the trash. It's okay though. Our relationship has reached a new level. We've officially pooled together our Pokémon cards.

For better or for worse, in sickness and in health, this place will be our unapologetic limbo where we eat, sleep, and incubate until something better happens.

It reminds me of my former on-campus apartment a lot. The one where I was shot.

LITIGATION II

I travel an hour to City Rehabilitation & Vocational Services, an apparent offshoot of Integrity Medical Exams that focuses on the enigma of the mind. They have me fill out the same form—we are not here to help you, sorry not sorry—which I return with a tongue-in-cheek thank you so, so much.

Unlike Integrity Medical Exams, people work here full-time. The staff of City Rehabilitation aren't doctors, nor do they pretend to be. Like the enigma they study, they go by the ambiguous title of rehabilitation specialist. I wonder which one of them drew the short straw and had to go to FedEx to print off the phony certificates.

Another "patient" is in the waiting room with me, a woman with unnaturally black hair and heavy eye makeup who walks with a cane. At one point, she tells the front-desk person that she has had over thirty correctional surgeries in the past six years. I think she's in the middle of a workers' comp suit. How many people must come through places like this? How many niches of misery exist? That the able-bodied never see, until age or accident forces the eyes wide.

I want to somehow help this woman and bring her some sense of peace. Jim, my therapist, has recommended a meditation exercise to me. He's got a spiritual bent to him but I don't mind it yet. *Bless me into usefulness*, I repeat. A mantra. I breathe in, pretending the air around me is polluted by all the world's suffering, and breathe out. That breath cleanses and alleviates the suffering in some way. I close my eyes and imagine several fuzzy black smokestacks floating around me, like a swarm of miniature charcoal drawings of cartoon sheep. I take a hit and try to absorb some of the woman's suffering into my body. Given the circumstances, there's a good chance we've gone through much of the same.

As I slowly exhale the fresh, suffering-free air back into the atmosphere, I feel calmer and I peek at the woman to see if it's working for her yet. She is busy filling out the scammy intake form. The more she fills out, the more her jawbone protrudes from her skin like a fossil being unearthed at an archaeological dig site. She is clenching. She shrugs her shoulders in defeat. This whole rigmarole is humiliating.

No dice, Jim. Here, the house always wins.

My Rehabilitation Specialist could very well be Seth Rogen but at the same time in no way could be Seth Rogen because the real Seth Rogen understands fun. He leads me to a windowless room that looks like the inside of the computer operating system Windows 95. Dull, dirty, old, and gray.

To determine how the hunk of meat behind my face has been affected by the events of April 7, the man gives me puzzle blocks and he tells me to recreate the shape in diagram 2b.

Choreographing nine cubes, each cube half white, half red, split into triangles down the middle, I make the trapezoid that I see in diagram 2b. Diagram 7a resembles the enemy ships from the hit 1979 arcade game *Asteroids*. As the timer clicks down to zero, I do not have as much success with diagram 7a.

"Wow, I really pooped the bed there," I say.

Again, this Seth Rogen proves himself only a look-alike. Not a trace of humor. No signature pothead laugh.

I automatically assume the whole place is bugged with hidden cameras and microphones.

On the paper tests, simple arithmetic turns into fractions and decimals, spelling starts with the word *Go* and ends in *Omniscient*, which I spell *omniecent*. I feel a little more confident with word pairings and definitions: an anchor and a fence both hold things in place. Or do they each contain things? That's not the worst answer, surely. Define *redivivus*. I swear they just made this word up.

I loved school but I do not miss standardized tests. I haven't done anything quite this rigorous in some time. Two hours into testing, I'm exhausted, encumbered by a number of headaches, but there is no liaison or patient advocate here. There are definitely no nurses. With what may test as the mental capacity of a sleep-deprived third grader, I shake my head and signal that I need a break.

I walk back to the waiting room and ruffle through my bag for a snack. The front-desk person stares at me with a numbing gaze, long and hard. I realize that everything I do is being written down. From the slightest scooch of my chair to the time spent rubbing my temples. The woman from earlier, whose name I discover is Nita, walks by, looking even more tired and distressed, muttering to herself, "What a world, what a world."

———

Before I can finish my protein bar, Seth Rogen corrals me back to a special examination room set up with switchboard machinery straight from the first Apollo mission. I am to simulate working as a receptionist for a manufacturing plant, fielding calls and completing While You Were Out slips, wearing hilariously oversized headphones that smell like cigarettes, while at the same time sorting mail alphabetically into a tabbed accordion folder. It is harder than it sounds—and deserves way more than fifteen dollars an hour, by the way.

The ringing starts and my heart palpitates. The recordings are the same two voice actors, a male and a female, with that marvelous Turner Classic Movie sparkle in their voice, talking too fast in their own period-correct way. Each new call, they pretend to be different people by slightly changing their accent or pitch.

Like Lucille Ball mismanaging chocolates down an assembly line, I can't keep up with the tasks, may soon have to eat them. I toss mail for Ziegler, James in the back of the folder, catching tidbits of the call that's come in, chicken-scratching vague notes like *Anderson Corp. wants to merge?* Each section I fill out is illegible and incomplete. I'm trying to do too much at once and therefore doing nothing right at all.

"Say, uh, tell Bob to meet me at the Gentleman's Club after work, will ya? His wife and kids won't mind if he's a little late for dinner, see." Yes, this outdated sexist info is also vital to my evaluation. I felt like I was in a gangster movie from the 1930s.

"Is Mr. Lewis there?" There is a pause, like a television show for children where the characters pretend to wait for the answer to be blurted out. "No? Mr. Lewis is not there?"

There is no actual phone. I cannot answer her. *What the hell do you want, lady?!* I scream to the back of my teeth.

"Agnes. Just say Agnes called. Mr. Lewis will understand," she says with extramarital undertones.

After Agnes hangs up, I conclude that nobody works at this place. Why is nobody ever in? What do they even manufacture? How do they make any money? How do they afford the Gentleman's Club? This is a company built on lies. Anderson Corp. should rethink the merger.

Afterward, I bump into Nita in the hallway.

"The phone thing? I know I did bad," she says.

I nod. I failed the sorting section. I put Ziegler, James *behind* the Z, instead of in front.

WASTE

It's Frozen Pizza Day. We plan for it, look forward to it, every other Thursday.

Anna and I get the cheap ones and then dress them up with our own ingredients. Onions, green olives, basil, garlic powder, and sometimes more cheese. Sometimes feta.

I'm chopping onions, bragging about working at a goofy pizza chain for three years in high school. Anna is doing the olives, bragging about her travels through the Mediterranean. We make faces and bump elbows, watching couples on TV argue about which house to buy.

"We could never be on these shows," Anna says. "We always agree on the same house."

Waiting for the pizza to cook, Anna and I diagnose this house-hunting couple's underlying relationship issues, which seem intense.

"He hits her," Anna suspects.

"He's a gaslighting narcissist!" I say, which is obvious.

They need more square footage, to be as far away from each other as possible. We cringe every time we hear the term *man cave*.

Siri, programmed to call me Pizza Boy, lets Pizza Boy know that it's officially Frozen Pizza Time.

The day we plan for. Look forward to. Every other Thursday. A tradition I take solace in now that so much of my life is out of my control, out of whack.

With a spatula, I slide the pizza onto a plate, and aside from a particularly cheesy olive that I know Anna would have loved, it's a successful transfer. Four fat triangles and it's ready to go.

Walking back to the couch, my foot catches a folded-up corner of kitchen rug and, bracing my fall, I launch the pizza, which lands toppings down, near Anna's feet on the living room carpet.

I get up, dust off my pant legs, and just know. I know exactly what she is going to say. I know exactly what she is thinking, how she'll react. I know it is my fault. She doesn't want it anymore. She is so fucking picky. A germaphobe, really. She will tell me it's not worth salvaging. I know all this, and don't want to hear a single word of it. None of this is fair but I can't stop it.

"Don't fucking say it," I say through gritted teeth, the firmness in my tone a warning. "Don't say a fucking word. You are so fucking predicable." I'm pointing at her. "I'll fucking eat it."

My fuse, that once could wrap around the earth twice, is now the size of a rat's tail.

I can't let this be a waste. A waste of time, all the prepping, the ingredients, the money. I ruined a good moment, a great dinner, our special day. The waste of it, the ruin of it, triggers an anger handmade by April 7. When I think about the night I got shot in the head by my best friend at school, I get angry, and I think about that night a lot, and also getting shot in the head by your best friend at school causes a whole host of behavioral and emotional shit, anger and outbursts and impulsivity being kind of up there on the list.

Anna's face turns hot pink and puffy.

"Put that in your book," Anna says. This is where she'd like me to put my anger.

For the first time, I explicitly want to blame Mark. I want to tell Anna, *It's his fault! Isn't it obvious! He is why I'm like this now!* A quick and easy excuse. Hell, it even has merit. But I don't say anything right now. We will have that conversation another day. We will talk about not letting Mark infect our relationship with any festering hostility. About how blaming him is just another way of keeping him close, and in our lives. Then I will apologize, and Anna will forgive me. *This is no longer on him anymore*, I will say. *It's on me. I'm really trying to get better; it will just take time.*

Until then, I grab a chair and belly up to the kitchen counter, near tears myself, and eat the pizza on Frozen Pizza Day, refusing to let a decent thing go to waste.

INTERVENTION

Mom and I weren't always two peas in a pod. You wouldn't know it now, but when I was younger, we liked to (emotionally) hit each other where it hurt—and we each knew exactly where it hurt most. She would take my guitars away, refuse to let me see my friends, and tell me to go to school to be an orthodontist. I would hide the batteries for the TV remote, threaten to go live with Dad, and insist on being a musician.

We argued profusely. We were actually good at it, welling up with anger and misunderstanding. She would lie, I would lie, and we would play those devil games. Our current relationship has grown out of respect for each other's stubbornness, among other things.

When she stopped dismissing me as an inferior decision-maker, and I dismissed the idea that loving one's mom is uncool, we could finally start getting along.

Mom asks me to meet her at Starbucks for a one-on-one. We order, and find a spot to sit, in the middle of the room on these hilariously huge lounge chairs. Are they supposed to create a sort of nostalgia by simulating childhood, when one was much smaller than their surroundings? If so, it's perfect for today's talk.

Mom takes a sip of coffee and says I'm different, says I've lost my twinkle.

"You're different, Paul. You've lost your twinkle."

Mom's feet can't touch the ground. It is hard to take her seriously.

She says my sisters agree, and Anna too. They all encouraged this meeting. They love me, and they care, and they want me to know they care.

"You used to be so lighthearted and patient. And funny," Mom says. She won't say what I am now. But by the law of inverses, I'm bitter, short-fused, and sad. I want to say, *Duh!* I want to say, *Fuck off.* I want to say, *Yes, I know.* Grandma didn't talk to me for months after April 7, afraid of how much my personality changed. I'm aware I'm not twinkling. I can't be happy all the time; it wouldn't be sane. I wouldn't want to be. That version of Paul is dead. I am a new person with old hobbies. I am 90 percent changed. A switch was flipped that day and has yet to be toggled back.

I liked the old me a lot better too. If we're lucky, he'll pop out every now and again, testing the waters, then maybe, as he adjusts, he'll pop out more frequently. But for now, you're stuck with the new me. Face it, there is a certain something I have to carry now.

I say all this to her.

She says she understands. But I really don't think she, or anyone, can.

My family sometimes forgets the whirlwind of stuff I have always swirling around in my head. Dents, damage, and scars. The Painful Game, invasive thoughts, and bad memories. Without a proper outlet, without essential closure, there is no safe place to put my anger. I have to sit with it stirring in me like a tiny venomous animal. A chimera that nips and claws, chews and erodes. Until I can't contain it any longer and it unleashes, misplaced. Stuck in a time loop, a trauma spiral, a cycle of assault, I become vile on behalf of the incident.

Everyone expects me to be better, but I'm not. The reality is that I may continue to hurt those around me as my brain heals and I relearn who I am with this healing damaged brain. I don't want to be a scary person. I don't want to be different in bad ways. I want to make a breakthrough.

Mom grabs my arm and says she misses her boy. I rub my face. I want to cry but hold back. I try to stay tough and in control. I think, *I don't need to be happy right now. I don't need a hug. I just want to be taken seriously.* That is the curse of the youngest child. Spoiled, yes. But a baby in the family's eyes forever.

Sinking into my oversized chair, I worry about potential eavesdroppers.

After a deep breath, we switch roles, and I become the adult.

"You don't seem too chipper yourself," I point out. I suspect things have gotten worse with David since I moved out. She makes no mention of him, but not even twenty-four hours later David will text Mom, in so many words, that he can't handle her life and all that she has going on. David was the first person to expect life after April 7 to go back to normal just like that. He was mad I didn't help around the house during my stay, mad after every meal, those damn dirty dishes. He knows he is being selfish. He says this. But soon enough, they split up. He will keep the house. Mom moves back in with Krystin.

But here in the big chairs she stays on message.

"Maybe you should try medication," she says.

"I already go to therapy," I say.

"Your sisters tried it and look how much it helped them. You don't need to take it forever. Just until you get out of this funk," she says. "You know we have a history with bipolar and depression."

This is a life-changer, not a funk. I tell her I can't be bipolar because when I'm happy I'm usually pretending.

"You should still try it," she says. "You are always thinking about what happened. Give yourself a break."

I give Mom a firm maybe. But in the back of my mind, I know my crater will never buff out.

BIRTHDAY

We were at Krystin's place, celebrating my birthday. We were about to eat.

A buzz pulsated from my pocket. I let out a hungry sigh, interrupted by an unusual notification on my cell phone.

I put down the fork so that what I had considered a perfect bite was suspended in air, like a log chute action shot, not a bit of runoff onto the plate.

That's when it hit me. Who would even want to talk to me on my birthday anyway?

April 7 left me alienated from everyone I've ever known. My college friends were lost to the day itself; not one had reached out to me since. My high school friends knew nothing about me, about this; hitting them up was impossible. I was afraid to leave the house. Afraid to stay out of the house for any significant amount of time. I was offline, thanks to my personal injury case, not one photo, not one update. My guitar videos had a very passionate, albeit, lean, following. But now I was totally off the grid. I had been disappeared. I died a different kind of death, consigned to the purgatory of waiting for a settlement.

I honestly couldn't think of one person outside of this room who would want my company.

I hadn't even been signed in. Thumbprint scans, security questions. And there, via Facebook Messenger, was a note from my elementary school gym teacher, Mrs. Thompson. Her profile revealed she was a member of some sort of Tea and Fairy cosplay society with other retired elementary school gym teachers; they wore elaborate dresses with polyresin wings. Mrs. Thompson had climbed the ranks all the way up to Fairy Queen, in possession of her very own throne and scepter.

Along with a photo of a dog wearing a hat shaped like a birthday cake, she wrote: *Wishing you a wonderful year ahead.*

She sent a second message.

Happy Birthday. Do you remember in 5th grade your class got a new student after the year started? He was home schooled and way behind where he should have been academically. Anyway, when he went outside to test the mile run, he yelled at me while sitting on top of the sledding hill and said he hated me. He was totally angry and out of control. You were the one who talked him down. It was one of the kindest things I've ever witnessed between two students. I think about him a lot. He was so maladjusted. Thank you for your words to him. You are one of the nicest kids I've ever had the privilege of teaching. Bless you Paul.

For months, I didn't know how to respond.

LITIGATION III

Nita and I are both back at CITY REHABILITATION SERVICES. I smile and wave first. She recognizes me after a second.

"I'm still surprised you're taking the tests," she says. "You're so young, I figured you worked here."

I say I'm in recovery from a bad accident.

"I haven't driven a car in years," she says. "I wish you the best of luck."

"Same goes to you," I say.

We're offered coffee for the first time, which we humbly accept.

Not Seth Rogen calls me back to another windowless room, this time like the inside of the computer operating system Windows 98. Dull, dirty, old, and gray, but less so than before.

We begin with vocational exams. Which wrench has the most torque: A, B, or C? Which way does the switch need to be for each lightbulb to run in parallel? Follow the schematic. I have no clue what any of this means and cross off electrician as a career alternative.

Next, a general knowledge *Jeopardy!*-like oral exam. Fun, right? Let's have fun measuring my brain damage!

Question 1: This is the most widely spoken native language around the world. What is English? Nope, talk about self-centered. The correct answer is Chinese, nimrod. Lacking a tacky suit coat and a superlong and skinny microphone, Not Seth Rogen makes for a terrible game show host.

Question 2: Who is Mahatma Gandhi? Clearly someone you people know nothing about, I say under my breath before giving my real answer. Which is, a civil rights activist. Not Seth Rogen says I need to be more specific. From India? He scribbles a check mark in his workbook. I guess that was the magic word.

Question 3: This is the largest organ in the human body. Isn't it something ironic, like the small intestine? There's no buzzer to ring in. I'm the only contestant, so I just blurt it out. What is the small intestine? Nope, wrong again. The correct answer is skin, which is creepy to think about.

I request a refill on that coffee situation between exams, followed promptly by a bathroom break. My startle response gets triggered in the hallway by the front-desk person, who, also on her way to the bathroom, used a secret employee-only back door that opened to my immediate right. I hop back, letting out a minor reactionary Midwestern "ope." To play it off, I itch the back of my head and try to force a smile without showing teeth, lips like two raw hotdogs pinched in the middle. But it's too late. I can feel my chest getting hot and blotchy. To gain credibility with the Rehabilitation Specialists, I cite this incident as evidence to support my claims. Naturally, it does not end up in the final report.

Following my snafu with the front-desk person, memory and concentration tests are administered, not unlike the occupational therapy assessment I was given in those early days post-surgery. Three new words to not remember. More money to mishandle. Different permutations of digits to screw up as I recite, first forward, then backward, then in ascending numerical value. There is a new simulated day to royally fuck up. I get jealous of this imaginary Paul, who is out running dumb, mindless errands and not stuck in a scummy, outdated strip mall being humiliated by simple test questions.

The kind folks at City Rehabilitation have a full day planned, but it's not like they're going to skip legally mandated lunch. The staff gathers around a circle table in the waiting room and let Nita and me know there's a Wendy's nearby.

In my car, I eat a turkey sandwich that's been sitting in the passenger seat for four hours, but in twenty-degree weather, so I call it a wash. By now, the medieval torture device that is my own head is set to High. I start my car for heat and the radio and eat my sandwich while staring at the BWM dealership next door. A few spots over, I notice Nita is in the passenger seat of what I assume is her caretaker's car, eating some sort of pasta out of a Tupperware container. I'm not exaggerating when I say that she is the closest thing I've had to a friend in years. I'd like to think I've helped her feel less hopeless and alone throughout this whole ordeal too.

In the afternoon interval, I'm administered a mood and personality questionnaire, consisting of over three hundred true-false statements such as: True or false: people will often lie to get ahead. True or false: wherever I go, I often feel like somebody is watching me. True or false: good and bad spirits can occupy people and make them do things.

For the first time, I feel like I know all the answers.

STRANGERS

For the third year in a row, I volunteered as an elf for a nonprofit operated by Anna's family. Her dad had bought a steam engine from a museum and spent years renovating it; the family runs excursions complete with historic railcars around the United States. This one— and the elf part may have been a giveaway—went to the North Pole.

Outdoors in below-freezing weather on a platform stage, I "made toys" on a workbench conveyor belt just outside of Santa's Shack. I tapped toys already made in China with a ball-peen hammer, wearing candy-cane spandex and a hat with fake ears stitched on either side.

The train would roll up, Santa would emerge from his shack, the only heated trailer at the North Pole, something Santa was very protective of, jolly and warm, then climb up the vestibule onto the train. A whistle would blow, and they'd chug away, leaving us out in the cold like separated lovers in a Tolstoy novel.

The last two years, I was a higher-ranking elf, a troubadour, playing guitar with Mark inside the toasty train depot. Higher-ranking elves get ties instead of spandex. We were a big hit, but if I continued the tradition without him, people would have asked questions. What's up, where's Mark? I self-demoted to avoid the answers. The two hunks of ice that were once my feet had me second-guessing my choice. It was something like negative thirty with the windchill.

I ran into one of Anna's cousins who I hadn't seen in some time. She made a comment about how long my hair was getting, which excited me.

"I'm trying to look more and more like John Lennon every day," I said.

An older guy walking past overheard this and poked his head into our conversation. He slid the frames of his aviator sunglasses toward the tip of his nose, looked me square in the eyes, and said, "The only thing you gotta do to be like John Lennon is get shot."

BASKETBALL IV

The Timberwolves are playing the Utah Jazz. The Wolves are losing 61 to 50 at the start of the third quarter. I'm wearing my aurora green Karl-Anthony Towns jersey, have been wearing it all day, including to my niece's Sunday School choir recital and brunch, where I made sure to tell everyone in the buffet line that it was indeed my Sunday best. The jersey is so obnoxiously green, I was hoping to attract other fans, a glowing beacon of hope among a sea of formal dresses and ties.

Commercial. Anna mentions that I've been way-sad lately. More so than usual. I never really relax. The other night, I beat down the dishwasher when a bowl got wedged in the drying rack, clobbering the interior of the machine multiple times with the very same bowl it refused to give up. Just now, during the first quarter of the game, I lifted the ottoman entirely over my head wanting to slam it back down to the floor. Over a shitty three-point closeout.

I shrug, ignoring Anna's comment. I have not taken Mom's intervention advice. I've not started any medications for my moods. I'm thinking about April 7 all the time, about the Painful Game all the time. There is no way for me to be reasonable about a bowl stuck in the drying rack. My life is a human-sized Chinese finger trap: the more force I use, the more I struggle, the more stuck I get.

Gorgui Dieng drags his pivot foot after a pump fake, travels, turnover. Donovan Mitchell shakes his defender and slithers to the rim for an easy layup on the other end. More than ever, I'm envious of the athletic ability. The sheer talent. The exceptional fitness. The success. The brotherhood. The pack mentality. I crave all of this. Their bodies will fail and rebel years from now, some sooner from injury, and I sit here knowing what that failed body feels like, what their futures look like.

Andrew Wiggins misses a point-blank gimme and I look seriously at the ottoman again.

Anna says, "They're so bad. Why do you keep watching?"

At the time, the Wolves have a record of 44–34, our best season in over a decade. A long history of terrible on-court play combined with habitual unluckiness regarding draft picks, front-office moves, general dysfunction—being a fan is a masochistic existence. But our numbers are substantial, growing even. We are a community, we commiserate together, we complain together, and this sense of community, right now, is a release valve from the crushing isolation of recovery. Watching games, I can gauge my mental progress. Ticking along the season, I ensure time is passing as my legal dilemma drags on. The Wolves keep my mind busy, keep my hopes up. Watching the Wolves lose by 24, which they will do today, is genuine relief.

I've explained this to Anna many times, but I say it again. "It feels good to have something to root for, especially an underdog. You never know when something good is going to happen."

"*Goddamn fucking team!*" I hear from a fellow fan in the apartment below ours, female and furious, barely muffled by our building's insufficient insulation. A testament to the above, I sit back, relieved.

RAIN

A source of mine from inside the University recently sent me a picture of a new installation on school grounds. Situated on the fourth floor of the student center, not even three hundred yards from my old room.

From the ceiling hangs an enormous gothic-looking umbrella. Black and classic, the segments resemble bat wings, with sharp points at the cutoff of each vein. Strung with fishing line running down these points all the way to the ground, are bullet casings. And on the floor, about fifty more casings, outlining a circle, as if a thin membrane had somehow repelled them all, like rain.

In a country that endorses and sanctifies gun violence, on a campus that has in very recent history experienced gun violence, the most public statement by the University on the issue of gun violence is a gigantic magic umbrella.

RAGE

My bones are sticks of dynamite, organs C4, and my skin is made from thin sheets of plastic explosives, ready to detonate on command.

I trip over the power cable on my way to the bedroom closet. A booby-trap that triggers some oil drums rigged to explode.

A flashbang goes off as I flick the closet light on. My headspace is momentarily distorted. With one hand cupped over my eyes, I pull the sleeve of a sweater off the top shelf. Its molecular properties meld with every little thing it's touching: suspenders with metal clips, swim trunks with plastic ties, oversized belt buckles. As the pile avalanches down, every hard edge imaginable hits me in the face before falling to the floor.

The liner inside my khakis catches fire as I slide my foot in. My big toe gets stuck, and I drop to the ground on instinct. I manage to snuff the flame by kicking a nearby wicker laundry bin.

I forget what sort of space I take up on my way to the bathroom and run my shoulder into the wall. I am still calibrating my new body.

Looking in the mirror, I see the wound brand new. I see the bullet strike, like I'm trapped in a GIF or in my own reflection. I see my body get tossed back. The mirror splinters around a perfect, penny-sized black hole. For the first time, I hear my skull break.

Teeth need to be brushed. Good hygiene is fundamental to victory on the front lines. I hate how the comb is sort of touching the bottle of mouthwash, so I palm the cabinet as if to break its nose. I go to spit and despise the sound of running water. I palm the faucet as if to break its nose, too. Every inanimate object has got me cornered.

Wearing a coat offers a definitive strategic advantage. I tug it from the hanger, but it won't budge. I give myself permission to use excessive force. The hook pops off, snapping, after one big heave.

I inch the door open with a knuckle, to check for a trip wire, with enough time to slam the door shut if need be. Someone has likely mounted a gun with fishing line wrapped around the trigger. I tap, two steps forward, one step back, until I get the All Clear.

The door must be locked before I can leave. I miss with the key once and am tased. The metal enclosure has a current running through it. For people like me, who fail and who are in a hurry. My second stab is true, but I forget which way it needs to be turned. I hear ticking, a slow beep. To the right? Wrong. I jab at the door as the beeps speed up into one long tone. It is the metal in my head, picking up frequencies invisible to the naked ear.

LITIGATION IV

In his office for a pre-deposition pep talk, my lawyer tells me that if my left arm got inadvertently mangled at a steel mill, the insurance company we are dealing with would try to convince me that I didn't really use it much anyway, on account of me being right-handed, so why make a fuss? My lawyer says that if one of my sisters died in a horrific boating accident, the insurance company we are dealing with would try to convince me that she and I were rivals since birth, so actually, I emerged victorious.

They are ruthless, wretched beings.

The insurance company has hired a proxy; that is, they outsourced a lawyer to handle their bidding in our case. I am to speak with him today.

We are meeting in the biggest room on the top floor, decorated like the lobby of a five-star hotel. Marble flooring, sculpted wooden trims, brushed metal finishes, and contour lighting that accentuates the rich color scheme of dark green and tan. There's a refreshment station where a machine can make you a caramel macchiato, or you can top off your water bottle with sparkling instead of still. Within forty-five seconds, I've got enough beverages to drown an adolescent mule.

The proxy is waiting with an herbal tea. A humorless man, his face is deeply sun damaged, his dirty blond hair brittle, and I guess vacation home along the sun belt. He looks like the cartoon idea of an evil twin. He has a goatee and wears glasses, but not very fashionable ones.

This is our first of many meetings. I shake his hand just this once, then we take our seats on opposite sides of a huge boardroom table.

He starts. He is deeply saddened by what took place on April 7, 2017, and today, he just wants to get to know me. He's good at this because, for a second, I believe him.

After a series of introductory questions—where I was born, how I grew up, what kind of student I was, did I play any sports, have a job, or partake in any after-school activities—Evil Twin asks about my parents' divorce.

"I don't think Mark had anything to do with that," I say.

Divorces are hard on every child, is his gambit.

I'm still bummed out about it six years later, but the life-altering trauma hasn't added to the depression at all, not one bit.

My lawyer gives me a look that seems to say, *I'll let that one slide, but try not to be a smartass the whole time.* The opposition may use that to say I'm wittier than ever, my brain has barely been affected at all.

I fold my hands as though in prayer, fingers loosely interlocked like Lincoln Logs. I make my voice as light and clear as a choir boy, a chime, and say, "No, I never needed counseling for my parents' failed marriage."

"Tell me about your relationship with your father," Evil Twin continues. "As I understand it, you gave your mother full custody after the divorce, and now he lives out of state."

"We talk on the phone nearly every day," I say. It's more like once a week, but I'm really hankering to get Evil Twin off the topic. Truth be told, my father and I have developed a great relationship as of late. He's drastically changed, for the better. Neither of us is the same person we once were.

A clean bill of health up till now, both mental and physical, is one of my surefire saving graces, something my lawyer and I lean on heavily throughout this whole ordeal.

Evil Twin finally begins a new line of questioning.

"I see here that brain aneurysms run in your family. Your grandma, aunt, and your mother all have them. Could that help explain some of the headaches you may be experiencing?" he asks, pen wet and eager to make note of whatever comes out of my mouth next.

I throw my hands up without thinking, so caught off guard by how they even found out about that. My face contorts with disgust. I am shaking my head, sending Evil Twin a steady stream of phantom "no ways."

My lawyer reveals to me later that, unlike his other clients, he was hoping I'd get mad during my deposition to help prove a point. The ease with which my switch is flipped is a benefit, just this once.

"They run on the female side only," I say. I feel dirty, playing defense like this.

"You know that for certain?" Evil Twin says, edging the pen's tip on his legal pad.

"Yes. My neurosurgeon told me so after he was up close and personal with my exposed brain." I get the smartass glare from my lawyer again.

Evil Twin strokes his goatee while reviewing some papers.

"What's the deal with this book thing I keep hearing about? It says here you are looking for an agent. Any luck with that?" He takes a sip of his tea, as if to say checkmate, but he burns his mouth instead. I cover my smile as Evil Twin snort-coughs into the back of his hand. It sounds dry and painful.

It always comes down to money. The angle here is that they think I'm trying to make beaucoup bucks off my injury. I'm not brain damaged and traumatized; I'm a cunning opportunist.

"I am a writer," I say. "I went to school to write. This is what we do. It helps me process things like therapy. My therapist, Jim, encourages me to write. I'm looking for closure wherever I can."

Then I think to myself, *How cute. These dudes think books make good money.*

RAGE II

On my way to the office, I'm convinced that every driver with their window down is looking to shoot me in the face as we edge up, side by side, waiting at a stoplight. Someone makes three similar turns as me and I'm sure they are a settlement agent, tailing my ass.

Yes, I can drive! Yes, I have a job! I still got shot!

In the parking lot, multiple people are just sitting in their cars. *To be in transit, to be in a car, is a transitional state, but you are here now! A parking lot is a terminal state. Get the fuck out of your cars and go to fucking work. Don't dawdle!*

From my cube, I hear people complain of migraines and past sports injuries resulting in knee surgery. Distracted, I mistakenly click the wrong document. Each conversation is like a little missile in the air.

"Shoot me an email."

"Gun to your head, ham or turkey for lunch?"

"Rearrange these bullet points."

"We need to pull the trigger on that proposal."

"Lemme pick your brain for a sec."

"I'm going to have to bring out the big guns."

"Know anyone who does professional headshots?"

"I don't want to jump the gun."

"We would really shoot ourselves in the foot if . . ."

"Yes, that's been beaten into my head since day one."

"No, stick to your guns."

"As things pop into your head, fire away."

"We are staring down the barrel of poor safety metrics."

"Get the young guns on that job."

"I really dodged a bullet there."

"Well, off the top of my head . . ."

"He's a bit gun-shy after that rejection."

"This article is going to blow your mind."

"They got me sweating bullets."

"We'll really be under the gun on Monday to hit that deadline."

"The drop-dead date for content is . . ."

"I need to be on this phone call like I need a hole in my head."

I stare at a blank sheet of paper for a while. Left temple is a blue wire, right temple is green. I have to rub the correct one in order to fully defuse.

A coworker comes by and says they enjoyed reading my recent blog post called "Permeable Pavements: A Green Stormwater Solution." It makes me want to crawl under my desk and jam a pencil into my thigh. I want to crack the cyanide capsule in my molar. While foaming at the mouth I'll shout, *Don't read those! They aren't me!* Then gurgle my way to the great beyond.

I go to the latrine to sit in a stall and de-stimulate. I can feel a cold coming on and promptly put some tissue plugs up my nose.

Certain colleagues are mad that I'm salary but only work four days a week. I want to explain, part my hair and show them why, share why I don't get sleep and need bathroom breaks like crazy. I thought I liked that people here didn't know. I'm at a disadvantage either way.

Quitting time. Back home. I am a primed grenade. Another chance to guess which way the key is supposed to turn. I'm wrong again, so when I'm eventually right, I practically blow the door down, shoulder-first, bursting in to live happily among the shrapnel.

I decide now is the best time to hang a small hand towel on the oven. It falls. I try again, this time forcing it into a tight blob, and it falls. I try to rip it in half but can't, so I throw it on a pile of clothes I plan on donating to Goodwill.

My body slicks up with sweat, turning red, burning. I'm brimming with dark energy. Every cosmic thing is working in opposition to me. *I'm* working in opposition to me. I clench my fists, flex my arms until I'm shaking, trying to force this incandescent rage out of my pores. Exhaust myself so I don't punch a hole in the wall.

Isolated and spiraling, in this moment, I explicitly, definitively blame Mark. Hate Mark. It's his fault. All of it. My pain, my PTSD, the case, the constant fear of my health deteriorating. He made this mess, now I have to clean it up. Again and again. What a shit deal. After doing so for years, I no longer desire to make excuses on his behalf.

I've become frighteningly akin to the thing that made me this way.

A human weapon, the epitome of violence. Senseless. Destructive. Lacking any sort of intellect, empathy, or kindness. Something that, if aimed at another person, could do serious, lethal harm. A rabid brute whose sole intention is to destroy, disregarding consequence.

I feel the need to inflict the same chaos outwardly that I feel on the inside.

I do not have a permit to carry my rage.

I should take deep breaths and count backward from ten. It is both trivial and the end of the world. It will be the end of the world again tomorrow.

I am the asteroid and the earth. Brace for impact.

PART III

CLEVER MORONS

Simply put, Mark got off on making people feel left out. He would go over their heads on purpose for a tension laugh, some phony superiority. But I was an insider. With me, his jokes always landed. Never over my head—right on target. I stuck with him, to him. He found the only true way to separate us. One has to laugh!

See us here, in line at the cafeteria, waiting for the next batch of popcorn shrimp to hit the heated buffet. Mark does his best to embarrass me, but I've learned his tricks.

"Paul, you gotta get those diapers out of the living room, this isn't a fucking retirement home."

"I get to wet myself right at my desk and never have to get up." There I am, playing along, accustomed to this spotlight by now. "When I wear them to class, everyone wonders why it smells like piss. Old building, I tell them. What do you expect?"

"Have you seen that new HBO special?" Mark asks, grabbing a cupcake.

"Which one?" Keith and I respond in unison. We ran through these same lines many times before. We knew the script.

"*Cowboy Butts Drive Me Nuts.*" Mark says it extra loud, for the seminarians.

"Volume Four?"

We were sophomoric geniuses. From the Greek words *sophos*, meaning clever, and *moros*, meaning moron.

Mark had this bit, going up to strangers, guessing their names. There we are, prancing, an equilateral triangle from a bird's-eye view, as he locks eyes with those who dared.

"Hi, Jake!"

"Good morning, Chloe!"

He adds friendly waves. He picks common, practical names.

We celebrate even the smallest reaction.

"Um, hey?"

"Hi, guy!"

"Huh?"

Not many people wanted to put up with Mark's shit. Sometimes, neither did Keith or I, but mostly we did.

We screamed bloody murder at the pavement as fellow unsuspecting students passed. The most curdling, phlegm-tossing racket. We put our vocal cords in a blender and pressed puree, now in the parking garage, blanketed with reverberation.

Provocateurs, us.

Mark loved the attention. I felt fortified with him around, as he coaxed me into situations I would otherwise avoid entirely.

Us in the elevator:

"Alex, my man, what's up?" Mark says.

Nope, not Alex.

"What floor?" Not Alex asked anyway, a common courtesy to strangers.

"Fire hat, please," said Mark, trying to trick the poor soul into pressing the emergency stop button.

Not Alex gave us a look of, *I just failed a test I didn't study for, dude, I'm not in the mood for any funny business.*

We crossed our arms, leaned back all cool against the backside of the elevator, and returned looks of, *Okay, geez, only joking.*

"Have you seen that new HBO special?" Mark asked us.

Keith and I always stuck to the script. *"Volume Four?"*

———

There is a single memory I have with Mark that remains pristine and untouched.

We were the Troubadour Elves, playing for Anna's family's Christmas Train to the North Pole. Mark, like all aspiring entrepreneurs, had a nonprofit, ran it with his dad, and I helped loop in this nonprofit to the event. Mark and Keith played guitar, Mark looking spiffy as ever in his surely expensive suit, Keith, who joined last minute, wearing an XXL Steam Engine in Christmas Lights T-shirt "borrowed" from the merch table. I played harmonica, wore my chicken-wire-and-duct-tape (a phrase my boss, Kate, would often say, referring to something cheap and hastily thrown together) suit from Goodwill.

After, our gang of four—the trio plus Anna—walked downtown to a nearby pub. It had been snowing all day. It was late. We threw snowballs at each other on the way, just like a cheesy Hallmark Christmas movie. Mark held the door open for us as we walked in. A few other train volunteers, rail fans in their late sixties, already had a table. We joined them for trivia, and they told stories about old train depots they worked at when they were our age, repurposed as coffee shops now. They were surprised we knew so much US history and we were surprised they were so much fun to be around.

Mark and I shared a batch of Korean BBQ wings and ordered the same lemon-infused lager. Each wing was equal parts the hottest and greatest thing we've ever tasted, even better than the last. He flirted with the waitress every time she stopped by. She seemed to enjoy his extraterrestrial sense of self while he played with the mucus that was dripping from his nose.

"I want her to sit on my face and use it as a toilet," he said.

Mark treated the world as his very own one-man play, where he had already won over the crowd and was now just biding time and enjoying it, even if something bombed. He could say whatever he wanted. There was an undeniable charm to him despite—or perhaps because of—his crudeness. If he happened to ruin a moment, you could chalk it up as Mark just being Mark. And that made it somehow okay.

This moment, notwithstanding using anyone's face as a toilet, was special, unlike any other. I did something extraordinarily rare: I took a picture of the full table, Mark's back to the window, Anna and Keith laughing together, the streetlamp outside a measuring stick for the snow. That night is forever bottled in sepia now. I hope Mark thinks of this day, looks back on it like I do, the rarity, the banality, the ease, the friendship. I hope he didn't take all this for granted.

We would have been each other's best men, groomsmen, bachelor party off the chain, bonkers reception. Undisputed if not for April 7. I try to imagine Mark starting a family, but it's hard. He preferred unserious relationships, dating app one-night stands; he staved off true emotion, actual closeness. Maybe the same could be said about his friendships. Though we shared some glimpses of tenderness over the years, I can't say I ever truly knew Mark. Most of the time it felt like all I got was the greeting, never let into the house. How much can you really know someone if they welcome you in so rarely?

Conversation returns to trains. There are only so many times you can rebuild a steam engine built in 1944. The train will end someday, placed in a museum, reassigned to history.

Mark gave the waitress his phone number—scribbled it on the check—but she never texted or called.

QUIET

Today at work, the coffee is everywhere. Someone must have tried to brew a fresh pot, but the carafe wasn't aligned with the nozzle. An entire industrial batch of coffee intended to serve more than sixty technical experts is now stewing on the countertop, seeping into the cabinets, and collecting on the tile floor drip by drip.

I should call up the St. Paul office to get in here, I think. The St. Paul office is home to our emergency response team who are cleaning up an oil spill right now, somewhere in South Dakota. I laugh out loud at my own joke.

Grabbing some paper towels, I clean the countertop. A water scientist walks in. I've edited his bio for a LinkedIn post, though we've never officially met.

"Whoa. That's a lot of coffee," he says.

"I didn't do it, I promise. I just walked in and inherited the mess."

"Whatever you say," he says. "I'm Brian. I don't think we've met. I've seen you around, but you always seem so quiet." Brian reaches his hand out for a shake.

Another person comes in; Lisa from the construction management team. She introduces herself. Like Brian, she's seen me around and noticed how quiet I am.

When they leave, it occurs to me that what Brian and Lisa are speaking to is something fundamental. They are trying to be nice, using the word *quiet*, but what they really mean is *you never smile*. You twitch a lot at your desk, in the halls. You're easily startled and we're sorry for scaring you. You keep to a bizarre time-sensitive agenda. You have not had a good night's sleep in a while. You're not friendly. You never make eye contact. You always look away. You walk with your head down.

I know for a fact one coworker thinks I'm perpetually hung over from some fantastical, never-ending bender of epic proportions. I go along with whatever people assume. It's easier. I wish I had the language to clarify my situation. The energy for some workplace bonding where I could explain that I got shot in the head by my best friend at school, but I don't.

For a change of pace, a sort of experiment, I try to not be so quiet in the hallways, just once, to see what it's like. I pick an air quality consultant whose desk is near mine. We catch each other by the water fountain. I say hello, ask him how he's doing. He responds with what day of the week it is, and calls me by the wrong name. I've been working here for over a year. This man passes by my cube at least five times a day, my name pinned on the prefabricated outer wall in a large, sans serif font for easy reading. It seems no matter what I do, I'll forever be the weirdo quiet kid from marketing. So why bother?

When I arrive back to my workstation, reassuringly disheartened, my boss, Kate, is waiting there for me. Probably wondering why I've been absent for so long, close to forty-five minutes now. I mentally prepare my response to any scolding.

"Paul!" Kate says.

"Coffee spill," I say, pointing my thumb in the general direction of the kitchenette.

"Yes, I heard," she says. "Brian and Lisa told me. That's pretty special you took the time to help clean. You really are the future of this company."

I internally cringe, but in remembering the pay and benefits package, a warm, welcome blanket even on my worst days, I contort my face into a smile and nod along.

Unlike with Mark, these mixed feelings are short-lived. I will be laid off due to marketing budget cuts in roughly six months.

TBI

This is not an issue book, in the traditional sense. It is not chock-full of data, statistics, bar graphs, pie charts. It is not researched in the way a book of journalism would be. *This* book is instead a living testimony, a gospel beyond the empirical, a story deeper than the standard news cycle, which hopefully makes it more meaningful. Something that lasts longer than twenty-four hours.

If I've been doing my job correctly, my views should be obvious without having to state them outright. They should be oozing out of every word. But I will formally articulate them now, nevertheless, for the people in the back.

Whether you are a gun owner or not, America needs major gun reform.

TBIs are no joke, especially those caused by gun violence. To recuperate anything resembling basic functionality—a new normal—victims require a special brand of patience and understanding, love that is unconditional and a sympathetic environment that fosters the goal: let's get better *together*. There is never just one victim when someone is shot.

At work, part of my job was looking for environmentally adjacent news stories related to our service line to share on social media. This practice exposed me to a lot of news, not just about Legionella in cooling

towers, or a new kind of pea-based alternative-meat patty. I started notic-
ing that TBI reports were just as alarmingly frequent as mass shootings:
a video clip of community protest, a call for gun reform all over social
media, some doom and gloom TBI article. Unrelated, yet not.

Parkland, protests, man who was shaken as a child dies from TBI
twenty years later; accidental school shooting death in Alabama, student
walkout day, child struck by tree branch in head dies five years later;
school shooting in California, general, never-ending Twitter Wars, baby
hit in the head with softball at father's game probably won't make it;
woman killed by stray bullet outside of Colorado restaurant; seventeen-
year-old dead after police shooting in public park; man walks out of
apartment building with shotgun and randomly shoots at houses along
12th Avenue; #GunControlNow, caption: *Boom! Boom! Boom! Students
describe the deadly scene as they listen to their twenty classmates getting
murdered.*

As expected, this was not good for my mental health. My mind can-
nibalized itself over problems it assumed but couldn't fix. It was far too
easy to obsess. I would wait for my turn, queued up to perish at the hands
of the TBI rulebook, any minute now.

When you know you're about to throw up and are on edge, abdomen
tensing with each quake in the back of your throat, helplessly afraid of the
body's autonomy, that was my existence around the clock. Lightheaded,
I'd often consider letting that take its course, a mercy.

FREE TACOS

I'm out with Anna and her extended family. We're sitting at a high-top next to a Build-Your-Own-Taco cart, which we're told is completely free to enjoy. I think the idea is that everything is so high in sodium, you'd get thirsty, and then to quench said thirst, you'd buy more drinks, which, in turn, would more than cover the food cost of the "free" tacos.

Anna excuses herself to the restroom to cry. Because of me, not this taco ploy. I don't mean to do this to her. I know the whole situation is depressing, I just don't want her to be totally shocked if she wakes up one morning to find my corpse.

I explain myself to Anna's family. About what I've been reading in the news, that I can't go a day without seeing my fate, the seizing, death from TBI, throw-up analogies, etcetera.

In short, they tell me this is no way to live.

Grandpa Gerry buys me a Miller Lite and says it's not what happens but how people respond that matters. In his point of view, I've responded with fantastic resilience. I wet my lips with the foam, just for a taste.

But I wasn't really listening. I was far off, somewhere distant. Thinking about my brain, the CT scan from my most recent checkup. Residual scar tissue, encephalomalacia, left prefrontal cortex. The areas around it will have to pick up the slack, my neurologist said. These parts of the brain are responsible for emotional stability, planning, abstract thought. I imagined that the scar looked like a Nike Swoosh. Pictured my brain contained in a half-filled snow globe against a black curtain. Cerebral fluid brushing up to it in little waves, like chemically treated water to a PVC pool toy. I smelled chlorine.

I stop myself before entering another Spiral. Grandpa Gerry just said it. It's not what happens but how people respond that matters. I need to make time for the things that matter, in protest, and carry on. I had to figure out my options. What could I do? What was the best thing I could do now? Should I do only ever exactly what I wanted to, every waking minute? Say, quit my job? That was tempting. Drain my meager bank account on courtside tickets to a Timberwolves game? Or a trip to Menorca? I'd only be able to pick one. There is no Make a Wish for people who are afraid they will drop dead at any moment.

For years after the shooting, I was encouraged to treat every waking moment as a gift. I took this platitude seriously, and it troubled me. If every moment was a graciously wrapped celestial package, I was mostly stomping each one flat to the ground when I succumbed to a bone headache, to the paranoia that hit with a guy parked outside of my apartment building, to the spells, the spirals. One hundred percent fun wasn't possible after gun violence or a TBI. What percent is? Forty percent? Seventy-four percent? Would it always feel like zero? Every day was a gift, and I'm the kid who asks Grandma for a receipt to trade it in for something better. The hurt on her face. Feeling horrible for it.

This new life came with limits and stipulations, with difficulties that guaranteed I could not enjoy every moment. It took me time to realize this whole gift business wasn't about simple enjoyment. Doing only what I've wanted to do, or what I've felt ready to do, provides little satisfaction. I'd give back this particular hardship in a second, but hardship is a purposeful, loving gift-giver that I've come to trust. A truly meaningful sense of accomplishment comes from challenging life's cruelest moments head-on, which is, apparently, the only way I know how.

Life is just a one-note vacation otherwise.

LITIGATION V

Halfway through my deposition, three years after the shooting, shit gets real. All my apparent delusions, my paranoias, my excessive Checking and Tracking, turns out to be warranted. I'm asked about it all.

Evil Twin asks me how often I leave the apartment, how often I go for walks, and where. He asks me how my social life is going, if I have any friends, or if I keep in touch with anyone from school. He asks me if my boss, Kate, thinks I'm a good employee, and if any such kudos have been officially documented. Every sheet of paper from HR that bears my name is directly under his nose.

Evil Twin asks if I ever film myself playing guitar, and if I ever send such videos to my family. He asks how often I play video games, and for how long, before I get a headache. I think, perhaps you'd care to know my shoe size as well? What brand of condom I prefer? Or what my favorite midnight snack is? We can make this fun if you want.

Every happening of my meager existence is invaded and dissected.

Evil Twin claims that my situation of working thirty-two hours a week is entirely preferential, and not disability based. He asks me, bluntly, what can't I do?

It's less what I can't do and more what goes on while I'm trying to do it.

Try concentrating on writing good, industry-standard marketing copy, sitting at your computer, typing, deleting, clicking, with the ever-present paranoia that someone is going to walk up behind you, put a gun to your head, and pull the trigger. Try concentrating on writing, say, a professional but not-so-flashy press release with a bone headache that, as you reach an hour without break, slowly develops into an eye strain headache hybrid. Try some harmless administrative task like posting conference attendee information on LinkedIn for coworkers who don't even call you by the right name while facing a meaty Spiral, because of this very lawsuit, in a shroud of unintentional secrecy.

I wish I would have said all that. Instead, all I can muster is:

"I am disabled! I am disabled!" My voice is a light shout, considerably distraught, as if trying to get someone's attention across a busy restaurant. I slap the table. My lawyer nods along, pleased as ever, as I flex my anger into shape.

Unmoved, Evil Twin takes off his glasses, diligently wipes the frames with a cloth pulled from his breast pocket, and switches gears.

"In your demand letter, it's mentioned that you didn't attend graduate school because of the incident," he says.

"Correct," I say.

"Did you apply?"

"No," I say.

"Did you take any entrance exams?" he asks.

"No," I say. What I forget to say is: I wanted to apply to several MFA programs. It's an entirely different process than other graduate school applications, more reliant on the quality of your creative writing portfolio and letters of recommendation. For most, entrance exams are completely optional.

"Did you apply the year before?"

"Yes," I say.

"Were you accepted into graduate school at that time?"

"No," I say. What I forget to say is: most people aren't. The acceptance rates for MFA programs are comically low by design.

"You probably wouldn't have wanted to go anyway because of the student loan debt, right?" Evil Twin asks. He smirks, half joking. But nuance doesn't translate well to a written transcript, like the one that's being typed up literally as we speak to be freely quoted in the event of a trial, without context.

"That's not true at all," I say. What I forget to say is: each one I planned on applying to was fully funded.

With each blundered response, I give Evil Twin more than enough ammunition to discredit my case. Nearing the end, I'm physically holding myself back from punching Evil Twin straight in the mouth, and yet the worst is yet to come.

Evil Twin asks me to detail what happened on the evening of April 7, 2017.

And I tell him. I speak the incantation out loud. With a lagging, languid rhythm, and the patient cadence of a public access TV voiceover. But halfway through, I weep uncontrollably. My lawyer calls for a break, which I use to vomit in a bathroom stall.

I resume, painstakingly recounting every impossible-to-stomach detail, and Evil Twin sits there like an insomniac watching any old three a.m. infomercial.

Evil Twin determines that I couldn't possibly have PTSD because I was blacked out for twenty minutes on the night of the shooting.

Evil Twin asks why I didn't call the cops after being shot in the head by my best friend at school.

I stare wide-eyed at the center of the table. My posture shifts rapidly.

"I'd just been shot. I was clearly in shock from an injury I could in no way anticipate. It was kind of an out-of-body experience. It was a nightmare, a living hell, and so I was just there. I turned into a ghost."

THERAPY III

I'm at a new therapy clinic. It's not that Jim didn't work out. He was great, in his own way. But Jim switched to a faith-based private practice that focuses on sexual purity. Not what I was looking for.

The waiting room has a miniature Zen fountain and fake cowhide chairs. Sleek gray walls, little twisted candies in crystal dishes free to grab. Sort of modern Bohemian. Someone always asks me what I want to drink. Everything smells like the skin of someone who just took their first bath after traveling the world. I think, *I should want to be that person.* But I find so much comfort in the familiar.

I'm called back into a room with a purple velvet couch that I imagine was once owned by Prince, and immediately spill coffee on it. I attempt to clean it up with nose tissues.

My new therapist, Emma, says, "No worries, this material is pretty easy to clean. So, what brings you in today?"

I tell her what brings me in today. She reacts how everyone reacts when they hear it for the first time. I tell her I'm interested in EMDR, and that my mom, who also works in mental health, referred me to her for her reputation of being great at it.

"What do you know about EMDR?" Emma asks. "Do you know what the letters stand for?"

"I'm sure I did at one point. But I totally forgot now," I say.

"Eye Movement Desensitization and Reprocessing. It doesn't necessarily have to be eye-related though. Anything that involves bilateral stimulation of the brain. We get both sides talking to each other, and work through the trauma with different visualization exercises. My job is to coach you through those, and help you stop if it gets to be too much. Otherwise, your brain does the rest," she says.

Emma runs through the different ways to get both sides of the brain talking to each other.

"You can tap on your thighs. But some people don't like that because their arms get tired. I can tap on your hands. But some people don't like that because they think it's awkward. We could do audio. If you bring headphones, a tone can play back and forth in each ear. Or you can hold pulsers, which are these little egg-shaped devices that vibrate like a phone on silent. The frequency and intensity can be customized to whatever works for you."

"The pulsers sound the best to me," I say.

"Perfect," Emma says.

I ask, "So what will happen? Is it like hypnosis? Simple and calming?"

"We won't really know until we try. But that it will be intense." She gives me an analogy: "It's like, say, your trauma is a trip to Florida. You can drive there or fly there. Traditional talk therapy is like driving there. EMDR is like taking a private jet. The increased speed will elicit a similar emotional and physical reaction."

Sounds like my ticket to Closure Land.

She says it might change how I remember that night, and the related events that followed. I say that might be nice. She says it will alter my feelings, produce some strong physical and mental reactions, but we won't really know the specifics until we try. She wants to make sure I understand this. I say sign me up. Maybe it will add some much-needed perspective.

To prepare for our first session, Emma says we need to get some base visualizations created. We also need to establish any known triggers.

Talking about triggers is even a trigger because of the word *trigger*. I ask if we can call them reminders instead.

"Yes, of course. Make a list of reminders throughout the week if you can. Next thing is, I need you to think of a strong mental container. We will store your reminders in there over time. It helps to start small. Will you be able to have a container by next week?"

"Yes," I say.

"Make sure it's strong," she says.

"Sure," I say. "I'll think of something."

"Once you figure out your container, I'll need you to think of three characters. Real or fictitious, to fit certain roles as we try to process your trauma," Emma says.

"Okay," I say.

"You need a mentor, a protector, and a nurturer," says Emma. "Do you already have something in mind?" she asks.

"I think so," I say. "The mentor is George Saunders, a well-known, award-winning writer that I admire. The protector is Geralt of Rivia, from *The Witcher* series. The nurturer is Mom."

"I'll have to really try and remember the name Geralt," Emma says.

"He is a Witcher, like, a mutant monster hunter, but inside he is just a big teddy bear. He has scars all over his body and can solve any problem," I say, explaining more than I probably needed to. "His hair is white, but he is not like an old guy. He has a silver sword for monsters and a steel sword for humans, who can be quite monstrous at times, as you know. Plus, he can do some light magic."

"Geralt. Okay, I think I can remember it now," she says. "Lastly, we need to create a retreat: A mental space we can go back to if the trauma gets to be too much. This also gives us a non-threatening way to test out the pulsers."

She hands me two things that look like eggs, one black and one gray. They are attached to some wires which are attached to a rectangle with dials. The rectangle is the size of a Game Boy Color. I grasp the pulsers like reins. We calibrate to my specifications.

"Can you think of a place, real or imaginary, where you feel the safest?"

I think of the best night of my life. A snowy night out to eat, after the Christmas train, with Anna, Keith, and Mark. A sepia-filtered photo.

"I have one, but Mark is in it," I say. "Keith and Anna, too, and some other people."

"Hmm. It would be best if you were alone. Say you and Anna get in a fight one day and you need to get into your retreat, she may affect its usability."

"That's a good point," I say. "I'll try to think of something else."

My guitar room as a kid always felt safe and warm and creative. I tell Emma about it.

"That might work," Emma says. "Describe it to me a little."

"It was sort of underground, in the basement, but had a window high up, by a ledge," I say. "Lots of guitar paraphernalia. A six-CD stereo, cool rug, and coffee table. I think a futon, or couch. Someplace to sit."

"Okay, let's try it. What should this space be called?" Emma asks.

"Guitar Room?" I propose.

"Okay, yeah, it can really be that simple," she says.

"Okay," I say, unsure if she's humoring me or not.

Emma says she is going to coach me into creating the Guitar Room. Then we are going to introduce my characters to the Guitar Room one by one, to establish their presence there, if needed later.

"Focus on a particular focal point in this room, or close your eyes if you feel comfortable," she says.

I look at the back of an empty chair with ornate curves. "I'm ready," I say.

"Enter the Guitar Room," Emma says. "Wander around the space. Explore things as you remember them."

I see the coffee table. With thick, chocolate-colored wooden legs and shallow chicken scratches showing its wear. Empty Dr Pepper cans are stacked in a pyramid on the glass top in an impressive double show of sugar intake and patience.

Sunlight is coming through the window above the ledge, setting fire to heavy dust motes while offering an opium heat. The room feels claustrophobic, but in a good way. The way a cat fancies sitting in a shoebox, pleasantly confined. Everything I adore is in plain sight. Everything I adore is in reach.

I see reds and greens and blues and purples and oranges in paisley on the wall. A poster of perm-era Eric Clapton brandishing his famed 1964 Gibson SG called "the Fool," a guitar that was hand painted by a Dutch artist collective of the same name. It depicts a nude cherub with a messy ball of hair oddly similar to Clapton's at the time, floating amid a tarot card–esque celestial backdrop, all colored in garish Day-Glo. There is a beautiful Dutch landscape on the pickguard and flames encircling the cluster of tone and volume knobs near the input jack.

"The single thread running through all my paintings is nostalgia for Paradise," the Fool's ambassador Marijke Koger once said of the instrument.[1] "It embodies hope for a better world with more joy, beauty and peace, whether it be in the mundane or on the 'other side.'"

I pick up the guitar I had at the time, a budget replica of the Fool, the instrument I used learning Cream's album *Disraeli Gears*, front to back, by ear. Wood and metal working in perfect tandem. Something organic mixed with something man-made, like me. Guitars have it figured out. I sell that guitar on eBay, the day after my fourteenth birthday, for an American made Fender Stratocaster in Sienna Sunburst.

"What do you feel?" Emma asks softly.

I touch my amplifier, easily the size of a washing machine. It is a limited-edition model that Mom bought me when she realized I wanted to take music seriously. I run my fingers across the turtle-shell-pattern Tolex and pay attention to the resistive texture, to the rings of coffee stains I've added on purpose, knowing they will make the amp sound more vintage somehow. It pairs nicely with the amplifiers' cream color. I can taste espresso and steamed milk.

My fingers stick the harder I press down, Tolex feeling like the underside of a clementine peel. I test the cabinet mesh too. I poke it, sink in to stretch the fiber weave until it's so thin, it's see-through. I feel the outline of four distinct, twelve-inch speakers. I pull back, and the mesh rebounds into its original resting position, like young, healthy skin. I feel suede, vinyl. Sprinkles of residual ashes from burned incense and the glossy front pages of guitar-store catalogs.

"What do you smell?" Emma asks softly.

I smell layers and layers of thin nitrocellulose lacquer, the goo used to finish guitars and make them shiny. It's an expensive process. It requires many coats. And it smells identical to Pillsbury Funfetti icing and cake mix. Cases and guitars reek of it. My fingers reek of it too, after hours of playing.

"Now exit the Guitar Room when you're ready," Emma says.

I nod.

"How did that go?" she asks when I return.

"It was good," I say. "Weird getting into it though. I felt like someone stuck a suction cup to my forehead and was trying to pull me into another dimensional plane."

"Oh," Emma says. "Want to try again?"

"Sure," I say. Worst-case scenario: I have a seizure or slowly slip off into death.

"Enter the Guitar Room. Notice things you didn't notice before. What do you hear?" Emma asks softly.

I hear notes wrapped in yarn, reverberating and echoing as if played in a canyon. They bloom in a slow, exhausted cascade, like adding dye to clean water. Drums keep time like a steam engine, with the occasional clash of thunder. I hear the songs of *Disraeli Gears*. I hear a psyche-delic, melancholy voice that sounds like a cello. The notes are so long they can't help but warble, trying to rope themselves back in. There are pops and clicks of overdrive, fuzz, tape delay, wah-wah pedals getting stomped on. The crackle of cables being plugged in and unplugged, adjusted, the pick attack on a nickel alloy string. I'm playing along. It sounds as if one could run an electric current through a shag rug and stained mahogany.

"Introduce your characters as you see fit. Let them come naturally," Emma says.

George Saunders knocks on the double door. I open. He gives a familiar, comforting Midwestern wave. Raising his right hand up as if to swear on the Bible, then nods his head and hunches his shoulders, as though sheepish.

"Hello," George says, coyly itching the back of his head.

I like his beard and glasses. He thinks this room is neat as hell. George reveals a guitar case he was hiding behind his leg. He brought his acoustic to jam, naturally. We play some American folk music and talk-sing the lyrics.

Geralt comes in through a portal and sits on the couch, armor and swords. He listens and admires, not saying much. Mom comes down from upstairs.

"Check out this song I just learned with George," I say to her eagerly.

She claps and then sits and plays a card game with Geralt on the couch.

"Your brain will tell you what you need to know," Emma says. "Exit whenever you want to."

THERAPY IV

Emma has asked me to practice a form of mental containment; that is, a way to separate myself from what happened. I am to visualize a strong vessel for my reminders. Like a bank vault, treasure chest, or safety deposit box. I see a toy trunk. No, a steamer trunk. At the foot of a bed, in the master suite of a nautical-themed inn. Probably in like, Connecticut or something. There is a white sandblasted steering wheel nailed to a wall. The walls are painted navy. It is forever early morning in this room, for me. Always a little cold.

The more details the better. Make sure the trunk is strong. Okay, the steamer trunk is old but the wood extra-sturdy, it's deep in grain, with lots of knots, and it's tinted gray from sea-foam. There are metal reinforcements.

It needs to be sealable. It needs to lock.

I picture a big-ass ornate pirate key with a cool skull, some wavy metal for sure. My laptop, too, appears on top of the trunk as part of the locking mechanism. Everything passes through a Word doc before it is stored inside.

Now, visualize yourself putting things that set you off into the trunk. Know that you can come back here and visit them if you wish. But that they are stored safety, no longer running wild. The goal is to remember them differently. To compartmentalize, living with them, not against them.

I put frayed carpet into the trunk. It passes through my computer and digitizes, turns to dust made from pixels, dust small enough to move through the keyhole.

I put pouches of chewing tobacco into the trunk. I put messy apartments into the trunk. I put leaning over into the trunk. I put navy-blue sedans into the trunk. Corners, walls, bathroom sinks, mirrors, the sound of fire alarms, the sound of doorbells, beds with call buttons, plastic food trays, hypoallergenic soap, medical robes, bandages, nonslip socks with rubber tread on the bottoms, loose clumps of hair, heads, scars, craters, lawyers, courtroom scenes in movies, insurance commercials, personal injury law commercials, and hunks of meat shaped like a fist, all into the trunk. Sensations: the cutoff of circulation to my feet, falling down, head rushes from getting up too fast, cold water running down my forehead, the urge to duck when something gets thrown toward me on a television screen. I put David into the trunk. I put David's house into the trunk. I put mass shootings into the trunk, but there are so many, it's hard to keep up.

I try to put Mark into the trunk. The upper half of his body refuses to digitize and turn to dust made from pixels. From the waist up, he is sticking out of the keyhole, twisted like a human tornado. I can't get rid of him.

CLINIC

Nearly a year post-injury, I had a milestone neurology appointment.

"Hi. Checking in for Paul. I have an appointment at 11:00."

The woman at the front desk makes a discomforting noise while looking at my file. A cross between an *oh* and an *ew*.

"Are you aware your balance owed is over $3,000?" she asks.

"Sorry, no," I say, as if I owe her the money directly. "This whole thing is from kind of a crazy injury. I should be receiving a settlement soon for medical expenses."

"There is a note on your file to call the business office," she says, clenching her lips off to the side. "Unfortunately, I have to call. It's my job."

"I understand," I say, full of understanding.

Cheryl, from the business office, sees here that the current balance owed is over $3,000. She informs me that a past-due notice was mailed weeks ago. That a payment hasn't been received in over thirty days. I try to explain that I'll soon be receiving a settlement to cover such medical expenses. I repeat the word *settlement*. Nobody believes in this settlement. In situations like this, even I'm doubting it. The bills mount, they come in like meteors, burrowing holes in the ground all around me.

Getting huffy, I add that my mom definitely set up an automated payment plan, a minimum payment once a month, like forty bucks, after we spoke to Jan in collections. I vaguely remember a Jan somewhere down the line, but for all I know Jan is my landlord or a figment of my imagination. But self-assured, I say, we set it up with her. With Jan. In collections.

"Yes, that's called a 'good face payment,'" she says. She continues to use this malaprop nonstop for the rest of our phone call. I'm leaning over the counter now, trembling, next to the doctor's business cards. A line forms behind me, everyone pretending not to pay attention, looking at the water cooler or the hand sanitizer, deep in thought, as if these are modern art pieces. Cheryl and I talk over each other incoherently before finally it is settled. I will pay fifty dollars today.

I hand the phone back to the front-desk woman.

"Fifty bucks," I say, defeated.

"Adding insult to injury, huh?" she jokes, an air of sympathy in her tone.

"You said it."

"This is why I don't work in collections."

In the exam room, Dr. B sits in his captain's chair and scrolls down his screen.

"Your records say you saw another neurologist?" he says.

I grow hot with shame. I didn't know neurology was a monogamous practice. I didn't know I was cheating.

I had harbored the notion, back when my life was an annual physical and maybe a visit for a chest infection, that doctors, as part of their practice, ensure that patients feel safe and comfortable. To diagnose and treat as best as possible. To encourage patients to get checked out regularly. But sitting in this room, with this doctor, I realize I'm building an aversion. I fear I'll avoid the doctor, unless something is shot-in-the-head seriously wrong, again.

"My lawyer told me to," I say, with my tail between my legs.

Dr. B looks at the floor and laughs without sound. In the end, Dr. B will choose not to contribute to the comprehensive medical report that we are compiling for our case, refusing to play in the Painful Game altogether. He thinks it's beneath him, my gut tells me. Doesn't want to get his hands dirty.

"So, what's going on?" he asks.

I tell him there are days I really shouldn't have gone to work. Days I couldn't get anything done, really. I tell him the prescriptions I am on, how many milligrams of each, what I generally took depending on which of the three distinct headaches I was dealing with. A different pill for the tectonic plate shifting pain, the genie-out-of-the-bottle overstimulation, and residual migraine.

I tell him I'm trying to get fit again, which he is happy to hear.

I ask why the back of my head still hurts to the touch. He says nerves can take a year and a half to two years to fully grow back.

I had no idea.

Then, Dr. B holds forth on dietary supplements; talks about elements on the periodic table; apologizes for nerding out; tells me I need to optimize my baseline cognitive ability; compares this to performance economy and horsepower; discusses the difference between a Prius and a BMW X3; references an episode of *Top Gear*; suggests I join an Ultimate Frisbee team; recommends melatonin; says I should be more social but does not address my general mental health; recommends a deep-tissue massage for my head but does not address the cost; informs me, apropos of nothing, that extra virgin olive oil has been known to shrink some cancers like melanoma when applied directly to the skin.

"It's fucking amazing," he says about the extra virgin olive oil.

He is the first doctor I've ever heard use the F word. Dr. B is thoroughly unhelpful but weirdly cool.

In the parking lot, I call Mom on speaker and hold the phone very far away from my head. We owe over $3,000, Cheryl doesn't know Jan, I might not even know Jan, is Jan a real person?

"I'm certain we have it on autopay," Mom says.

"That's what I told them," I say.

Mom double-checks and discovers she set up a payment plan with a different clinic that has a similar name. We, in fact, haven't made a "good face" payment in over thirty days. She transfers money, sets up autopay. There is no reliable timetable for a settlement. This well is running dry.

THERAPY V

The front-desk person highly recommends I pay one hundred dollars before leaving today.

"This whole thing is from kind of a crazy injury. I should be receiving a settlement soon for medical expenses," I explain.

"Couldn't it still be quite a while until you collect?" she asks.

"It happened last April, about a year ago. I have no idea. Probably soon?"

I ask if they take cards. Of course they do.

My first EMDR session begins out of pocket.

"Okay," Emma says. "We will start with your first target. You on the ground, looking up at Mark who is coming out of his room, in the hallway, with his hand over his mouth and a gun in the other."

She hands me the pulsers.

"I want you to think about that moment. Think of the physical response your body had then, the physical response your body is having now, and how that makes you feel. Connect the emotions with the sensations."

It hits me that EMDR is like those simulation machines in *Total Recall*, except the memories are yours, they're real, they're traumatic, and instead of having fun, you end up with a full-body version of erectile dysfunction.

222

I remember the on-the-fence feeling. *Man, Mark, I wish you didn't just shoot me.* I remember the pressure in my head, the determination to stand and look in a mirror. The quicksand sensation. The feeling of blood on my nose.

"I'm ready," I say.

Emma turns on the pulsers.

It hits me that EMDR is like a Plinko board where your brain is the falling ball and the slot it ends up is the resolution you didn't know you needed.

I close my eyes. My brain is firing off little twitches and movements. Neck kinks, wrist turns, elbow kicks out. I see Mark. He has already shot me once. He comes closer and shoots me seven more times. He then pulls me up by my hand and gives me a hug.

My throat is a handyman's level, with that little air bubble choking everything up. *I'm so sorry*, Mark says. *I'm so sorry*, like a prayer. *I'm sorry.* I'm going to pass out. Emma's voice brings me back.

"Something happened that didn't really happen," I say.

"Interesting," she says. "What was it?"

"He hugged me," I say. I can't say the rest.

"Okay. Let's go back. We want to treat these moments like squeezing a lemon. We will squeeze over and over again until we have all the juice out. Meaning, we will try to hit all the avenues of thought your brain wants to go down," Emma says.

I go back. To the kitchen island. How do I feel? *What* do I feel? Keith is frustrated. Mark is scared. I am sad, and passive. I'm twitching again. My eyelids feel very heavy. Attached are one thousand fishhooks towing five hundred bags of sand. I lie in bed. The cops come.

Mark says he has a permit to carry. The news emphasizes he has a permit to carry. Everyone knows he has a permit to carry. Would he have gone to jail if he didn't have a permit to carry?

Emma pulls me out.

"What happened this time?"

"I'm actually not okay with the lack of accountability," I say.

Something I've always felt but can finally put words to. "I don't want to be the reason he gets in trouble. I really don't. But . . . nothing?"

"How does that make you feel?" Emma asks.

"It hurts. It hurts that the University didn't consider my feelings when they let Mark graduate." Any punitive scrap of my closure remains unfulfilled.

Emma says that it's natural to feel that way. But to really move on, I can't want impossible things. External, superfluous things. I can't go back and make April 7 never happen. I can't change what Mark did. But I can try to change myself, from which little boomlets of positivity could fractal outward and snowball to something greater.

"This was also about the time I blacked out, so I feel very tired," I say.

"Your body tends to mimic what was happening in the past," she says.

The battery for the vibrating pulsers dies, so we revert to manual. I put my hands on a small circular table, palms down, so she can tap on them.

"When we originally set up your targets, you said the surgery was probably a nine, ten being the worst," Emma says. "Do you want to try to process the surgery now?"

"Sure," I say.

"Great. Think about the sensations and images from the surgery. How does it make you feel in this moment?"

"Nauseous," I say. "I'm fine with over-the-top gore in games and movies, but hyperrealistic gore makes me sick. Like torture gore. I'm very squeamish. Up until April 7 I had never even broken a bone. I'm still squeamish at the thought of breaking my arm right now, after everything," I say.

"Once you have those images paired up with that feeling in your stomach, let me know. There is a trash bin to your right by your foot if you need it. Don't be embarrassed if you need it."

I threw up during *Red Asphalt 2* in driver's ed class, so she's not wrong to assume.

We squeeze the lemon on my surgery. Emma taps the tops of my hands, alternating in one-second intervals, for two minutes at a time. We perform many quick sessions. We are having a séance of memory. She is the medium. She is either cornering the Ghost of April 7 or inviting him to come out and play.

I scoot around on the purple Prince sofa like a dog that can't get comfortable. An itch on my collarbone is insatiable. I need hind legs to scratch at it, since my hands are busy being tapped on. My breathing becomes shallow. I'm unintentionally holding onto my exhales. I wonder if it's because in this moment of my surgery a machine was doing the breathing for me. Emma pauses our work when necessary; she has me pretend to blow through a straw, so I don't pass out.

Our hour has come and gone.

"Before you go, let's enter the Guitar Room. We should get you to a baseline, slow your heart rate a little."

I say hi to Geralt, George, and Mom, then listen to a few minutes of my mind's interpretation of "World of Pain" by Cream.

Emma reminds me what we just did is very abrasive on the brain. She says I'll be emotionally raw for at least three days, extra susceptible to my triggers, or, er, reminders. We will start with this again next time. Keep squeezing the lemon.

I pay the front desk a hundred dollars and see Mark's navy-blue sedan on the way home. Probably not his, but the same make and model. My mind goes straight to the trunk. Are there guns? A guitar case for the semiautomatic?

My eye starts watering but I'm unsure if I'm crying, or if I just haven't blinked in a while.

I make it back to my apartment, drink a full pot of coffee, and watch stand-up comedy on the couch until I fall asleep.

LITIGATION VI

The insurance company has required that Anna, Mom, Krystin, and Alyssa sit for depositions. All four are to be done on the same day, with an approximate one-hour run time, each. It killed me to ask. I didn't want to bring my family into this. But they were always in it, from the beginning.

One by one, my family members enter the hotel lobby room on the top floor of my lawyer's building. They marvel at the coffee machine and text me what they've picked to drink.

They are each asked the same basic questions to start. Who are you? What do you do for a living? Where were you when you found out? How has he changed? What are his symptoms?

"Wherever we go—the movies, out to dinner—he is worried about an active shooter. He falls apart in crowds of people."

"Not only have I heard him wake up screaming from nightmares, but I had to get a bone graft for my back tooth from clenching my jaw while I sleep. We are all hurting after what happened."

"My husband's bachelor party? Uh, they went on a fishing trip. The boat only went one mile per hour. He didn't even drink at my wedding. No, sorry, I can't quantify how much fun he had. I was busy getting married."

"Considering I work in the mother/baby center, the brain really isn't my area of expertise. I'd rather leave any prognosis questions for his neurologists. Listen, my brother was one of the most brilliant young men I have ever met in my life. The way he used to write music and play his guitar, he was completely self-taught, always showed me he had the potential to do many great things. That was all taken away from him in a heartbeat."

I can't stress enough the profound flaw of personal injury litigation. Mine is but one case, but it is emblematic, I believe, of victims and their experience. I'm not special. I am the standard. A legitimate victim with a reasonable, justifiable claim, whose case wasn't ever going to be reviewed with impartiality and afforded due respect, but rather whose case was misshapen and distorted by a corporate entity, an insurance company, whose purpose is profit and minimizing loss. Blaming the victim is the bread and butter of their business.

It is unfathomable to me how anyone can participate in this business, but most of my story is unfathomable.

How were we to move on from this when we were forced to think about April 7, forced to retell April 7, forced to feel April 7, over and over and over again, by and for representatives of a system that is built to dehumanize and devalue the human beings involved?

Trauma victims are retraumatized all the time and, let me tell you, it feels personal. It *feels* that the other side has already won, in the pocket of the favored side. It *feels* they are actively, willingly trying to hurt you and the people you love. The calculated delays, the gamesmanship, the bullshit cottage industry that enables winning results. It *feels* insurmountable. It *feels* almost *fun* for them to topple on more trauma in the place of retribution and closure.

I can't help but take it personally. I was being punished for getting shot in the head.

LITIGATION VII

If it's not blatantly obvious by now, getting compensated for a gunshot wound to the head is not a cut-and-dry endeavor. No happiness is pure happiness with the case looming over, no end in sight. There is a cap on my well-being, my joy, and not only does Mark's insurance company know this, Mark's insurance company is counting on this. Every moment is numbed by the threat of a trial. A threat that only increases over time.

Mediation is on the books today. Pre-trial tomfoolery. Held in the hotel lobby–style room on the top floor of my lawyer's firm. We cannot go to trial. My mom texts me: your lawyer needs to do whatever it takes not to go to trial.

A hot iron is poked through my chest.

Neither I nor my lawyer have that much power at this point. Only one entity can make it happen, and I don't think they're in much of a hurry.

The mediations all go pretty much the same way. I grab a drink or three from my favorite machine in the world, and we begin. My lawyer, his paralegal, and I take our seats around the huge boardroom table. Evil Twin and the insurance company adjuster, a middle-aged man who once laughed in my face over video call, are down the hall in a separate room. A mediator bops back and forth between rooms, sometimes giving a spiel, sometimes receiving one, with the objective of a peaceful and satisfactory resolution for all.

The nerves always hit the same way, stemming from optimism but settling into fraught and leery, knowing that a simple "not today" could mean as much as another year until we can try again. My body tremors with a consistent, low-grade current, as if I have a retractable power cord in my wrist plugged into the nearest wall outlet. To counteract the shaking I need a dude out of nowhere to pop out and blow-dart a horse tranquilizer in my neck. My face melts as I nod off, slipping into warm, gooey rapture, until the voltage in my arm kicks up again and I feel like I could stay awake for a thousand years. My body fights itself in a tug-of-war over consciousness. It never gets any easier.

Today's mediator's name is Roger. Roger cannot believe this shit is still going on. Finally, I feel like a real mover-and-shaker is in our corner. My lawyer chats him up for five minutes, lets Roger know which aspects of our case are the strongest, something a jury would surely respond to, and then sends him on his way to the dark side, where he spends forty-five minutes to an hour. Maybe time moves differently around bad people, who knows. What I'm saying is, there is a lot of waiting, and not much action as one would think for something that takes an entire day.

I periodically glare at the door, trying to telepathically send Evil Twin and his companion a cold shiver or two.

During the downtime, I drum on blank notebook paper and think, *They are talking about me. Not thirty feet away, they are debating my life, its value. This could all end today. There is a real possibility this could end today. Or not. Please, God, let it end today.*

Over the span of these mediations, I jot down exactly one note to myself:

Evil Twin is a Fuck.

In major need of distraction, I talk my lawyer's ear off about hypothetical Timberwolves trades, and he updates me on the status of his kitchen renovation.

Eventually, Roger comes back to us with a shrug and a look of deep frustration. Little to no progress has been made.

"Well, looks like they reached the value they were authorized for today. I don't think they're going to budge," Roger says.

The cinder block tied around my ankle is kicked off the ledge, and I fall back down my pit of misery and despair into oblivion. I scream, but only in my mind.

My lawyer tries his best to offer me hope. He can tell I'm starved for it.

"We made progress. We knew they would do something like this. They are harder to work with than other insurance companies, but by and large, this has been going by the book."

In total, there will be five mediations. They will span almost four years.

SETTLEMENT

I'll admit, it's hard to put a dollar value on things you can't see. The effects of brain damage and trauma largely happened behind closed doors. They never saw me drop things I should've been able to handle easily, walk straight into walls, struggle to find a word that I've known since grade school, or encounter a meaty Spiral at the local shopping establishment. Instead, they saw me upright, driving, going to work, alive. I talked their ears off about all my symptoms, but in the end, they only wrote what they wanted to in their reports, free to exaggerate, speculate, and flat-out lie. One B-list physician wrote that my tendencies toward paranoia were most likely present prior to the shooting, and that now they just so happen to come in a specific flavor, so to speak. I met with this man one time. We spoke for twenty-five minutes. Yet he'd have you believe he was the one who cut my umbilical cord fresh out of my mother's womb.

It is easier to put a dollar value on the injury itself, as my lawyer did. Add up my surgery, chronic headaches, and strangely, the thoracic outlet syndrome I developed in recovery from chronically trying to protect my head.

With these amounts in mind, and a conservative estimate of my subjective suffering, my lawyer developed a range.

How strange to think a certain insurance company had committee meetings in boardrooms, rooms they reserved solely to talk about me and my injury, where adjusters made counterpoints and debated what happened, my prognosis. I can't help but relate this to old white men debating women's reproductive rights. It's laughable. What do *they* know?

My settlement would not be the be-all and end-all. No amount of money could close my wound, but it would be a start. It meant I could pay off debts that have added to my stress. It meant I could pay for ongoing medical expenses. It meant I could invest in myself and explore opportunities to contribute meaningfully to life. It meant I could purchase things that would help me cope, like a nicer place to live, a new guitar, or an actual vacation.

Most importantly, and I couldn't even begin to fathom the sheer delight of this reality, it meant that the Painful Game would be over. I would be free. In seconds, a good chunk of my paranoia would just poof out of existence. No more bogus doctor visits. No more panic attacks. No more looking over my shoulder at public parks, restaurants, my own bedroom. No more ghost-like online presence, unable to network, connect, or share, which is so vital for the work I want to do. No more fear of missing out.

I would reenter the world of the living, battered, but renewed.

Think of the amount that would be enough for you to agree, willingly, to be shot in the head. You survive, you live a meaningful life. But shot in the head. Think of the amount. Think of the amount that would be enough for you to agree, willingly, to endure the lifelong symptoms of a brain injury. You survive. You endure it. But trauma and disability.

I can say with absolute certainty that any settlement is nowhere near the amount any of us come up with.

LITIGATION VIII

A trial date has been set, even though we are going through the motions to avoid said trial. Nearer and nearer to this date, I enter a meaty Litigation Spiral. I sit cross-legged on my bed with all the notes, reports, charts, and photos scattered around me. The amount of space they take up is frightening. My stomach drops as I fall through April 7's trap door, repeatedly. The pit seems hopelessly deep today.

I'm waiting for a phone call from my lawyer, who is waiting for a ruling from the judge assigned to our case that could change the boundaries, change all the rules of the Painful Game in the worst way. During the motion hearing, Mark's insurance company, led by Evil Twin, proposed that since Mark is admitting guilt outright, we shouldn't be allowed to talk about anything that happened in the two hours between the shooting and when I am taken by emergency services to the hospital. No running to the parking garage to hide guns. No lying to Public Safety. No thinking about a quick trip to Home Depot for plaster and paint. No bumming around the kitchen island doing nothing. Nothing. None of it. Evil Twin says this would be prejudicial, and thus the damages would inflate beyond reason.

This is what happened. How can we not talk about what really happened? Where is the fairness in that? If a jury ends up hating him, that should be their right, right? Well, no. Evidence is debated in cases all the time. A trial is not made of all the collected evidence. It's made of what's admissible.

Essentially, the judge is deciding a few things:

If this evidence is even necessary—there may already be sufficient evidence for a jury to fairly come to a verdict.

If this evidence is inflammatory—damning such that a jury would be blinded by emotions and rendered incapable of fairly coming to a verdict.

It is the judge's task to weigh evidence against emotions.

I run through the indisputable facts, shuffling through my own emotions and various physiological unpleasantries, namely tremors, increased heart rate, and throat tightening. I imagine grabbing Evil Twin by the lapels and screaming in his face.

To prepare for the worst, I make plans to dissociate through my would-be trial. I will sit in the courtroom and listen to countless lawyers, doctors, neurologists, and psychologists debate every aspect of some pretend dude's problems, past, present, and future. Can't be me. I'm calling it Codename *Dateline*, which Mom and I would watch every week when I was really little, snug on the couch together, sharing a blanket, way past my bedtime, with the biggest bowl of popcorn and chocolate-covered raisins.

Episode after episode, it wasn't so much the dismemberments, bloody crime scenes, or police interrogation mind tricks that fascinated me. I was always left pondering: What do these innocent-until-proven-guilty murderers do in the months leading up to their trial? If they make bail, do they just go about their normal business, cool as a cucumber, quietly walking among us? A trial is something I simply cannot handle emotionally. The average human isn't built for it. Maybe the murderers are. Good for them. I really mean that.

———

My lawyer calls. The judge has ruled we can talk about select details from that crucial two-hour window. In her write-up, much to the dismay of Mark's insurance company, she says, "Imagine this happened in a parallel world where Mark receives help immediately. I find it reasonable to assume that Mr. Rousseau would not have the same level or intensity of psychological traumas. Perhaps his headaches, too, could have been more preemptively treated if acted upon earlier."

THERAPY VI

Emma asks me to reveal one truth I know, with certainty, about myself. I say that's a tough question. My brain says: *I got shot, I got shot, I got shot, I got shot, I got shot, I got shot.*

I get up, take a few steps forward, toward my room, pause, turn one hundred and eighty degrees, face the couch, and lean over to grab something off the floor. A split-second decision to clean. Perhaps a scrap of paper caught my eye, or a dead battery, or guitar pick. I don't hear it. I don't see it. But something comes at me through the wall.

I feel blindsided, tackled into a pool of cough syrup. Soaked in thick liquid while wearing layers of yarn. My ears buzz as if someone hit the monkey bars with a tree branch in my brain. The sensation becomes a chronic, caustic companion. I lift my forearm, which now looks and feels like an hourglass. My sight is a television color quality test. I hoist myself up, without thought. I tell my legs to move but they stumble as if they forgot how. I am missing my steps, evaluating the depth of the floor all wrong.

But I get up. I keep trying, no matter the setback. I consider all I've managed to accomplish since that day.

"I think I'm strong," I say. "Not like in a bodybuilder way, but you know, I think I'm pretty resilient."

"Yes," Emma says. "I think you are the most resilient person I have ever met."

SETTLEMENT II

My personal injury case officially settled via teleconference on March 30, 2021, amid the COVID-19 global pandemic. Three years, eleven months, and twenty-three days since the shooting. Just a week shy of the four-year anniversary. The process was so soul crushing, I'd be lying if I said I never felt like giving up and ending my life a few times throughout. For whatever reason, admitting that comes with great relief.

A silly judge's ruling didn't make Evil Twin throw in the towel. If we thought that, we'd be forgetting everything we know about insurance companies. After the judge ruled on the pretrial motion, the insurance company decided to hold a three-month-long, $50,000 mock trial in front of a focus group, where they tested various versions of the case against those who identify as fiscally liberal, fiscally moderate, and fiscally conservative. Those results finally pushed them over the edge. I'd love to meet whoever played me.

The day the check came, my lawyer texted: *I've never had a more deserving cause or client. Thank you for letting me and my team be a part of your journey.*

I legitimately broke down from that.

I was close to having second thoughts about it being over. By that I mean, it felt like leaving a cult, its leader tricking me into believing that I couldn't live without them.

Due to the nefarious alchemy of trauma, April 7 froze me in a barely habitable stasis of suffering and woe. After feeling like my humanity was an insurance company asset for so long, it was about time to move on and be the sole proprietor of my future. The emotional toll of the Painful Game made me even more hardheaded than before. I felt like I could take on the world, in any capacity, and that nothing could intimidate me.

FRIENDSHIP IV

Keith, Mark, and I are still collected around the kitchen island. I realize something horrible. I know they are thinking it too.

Take everything in, friends. This is the last time we will all be in the same room together.

How can you come back from this? You can't come back from this. You don't.

Standing in the exact same spots before the shooting, we had once placed bets on who would make the most money out of the three of us. Who would get arrested first? Who would get married? If dorm-room veneer could speak! In the time it took for a projectile to muscle through a few walls, all of that ended; all bets were off.

An invisible line is tethered to me and that old apartment forever. There is residual energy, an echo, a manifestation, a haunting.

Losing Keith and Mark was losing my five senses. I was robbed of the primary way I perceived the world. They were my cues, my context.

I had lost my limbs. I was unmovable, abandoned, marooned, living on the speck of Brain Injury Island, population one, isolated, aching for phantoms to help me find purchase on the earth.

It was forgetting a birth tongue. We spent years developing a language based on arcane meme references, inexplicable social cues, and postmodern cringe comedy that each of us will never be able to speak again. Keith and Mark were the physical embodiment of the voices in your head saying things you wouldn't dare say to your parents.

Like most friendships, ours was born from convenience and proximity, by chance. Think neighborhood kids, with nowhere else to go, flocking to each other's houses for no reason other than that we were the same age. Mark and I didn't choose to live across the hall from one another. We were complete strangers, with very little in common. Our similarities and connections were shaped by cultural trends, the time in which we lived. Our friendship was easy. It fell into place and found a groove. Call it naivete. Call it the shimmering privilege of youth. But I rode that groove, gleefully trucking along while I overlooked red flag after red flag.

We aren't always attuned to red flags, or maybe we see those flags more orange than red, because we understand humans are complex, complicated, flawed. Sometimes we do see these red flags but far off in the distance, barely fluttering, because in our full view, we're seeing good things in the foreground, appreciable and valuable things, and that's where our eye sticks.

Mark preferred irony to honest emotion. Our relationship was never what I wanted it to be or what I really needed: something unmistakably true, something so sincere it hurt, something real. I knew deep down that no matter how integral he had seemed to my very being on a daily basis, I had never been able to depend on Mark in any emotionally significant way. In any way.

Friendships end for all kinds of reasons. People grow apart. Invisible grievances crop up. Values change. Some special fulfillment is no longer met, by one party or the other. People find all sorts of ways to not need each other anymore. It is a shame that my friendship with Mark never had the chance to either end on more conventional terms or grow into something more meaningful as we matured and experienced more of life. Instead, my time with Mark ended with a bang and splintered from the force, revealing it to have been a thin and brittle thing all along. Some relationships are simply not built to last. Not everything that breaks needs to be repaired.

I've separated myself from the violent end to this friendship. The hard work I've done in therapy and through writing has been a powerful neutralizing agent. Mark's grasp on my life has weakened over time, and I can safely and confidently say that all these years later, I can't locate his hold on me at all.

That he is to blame is a fact. He is responsible for what happened to me. He brought the gun into our apartment. He pulled the trigger. He failed to take action, refused to take immediate responsibility.

For a long time, Mark held power over me simply because I clung to all that resentment and anger, let it fill me to the brim. I've slowly but surely let those feelings go. This requires giving Mark zero real estate in my head. And if he pops up—as he does, as he always will—he doesn't stay very long. I move forward. I am revitalized in body and living the best I can with my own senses, my own limbs, my own language. Mark is just one thread of my story—one essential, motivating, unavoidable, crushing thread—but the whole of it, the heart of it, is the moving forward.

YEAR

It's exactly one year post-shooting. I'm calling April 7 my second birthday from now on. After hyping it up for a few weeks, the family has
followed suit. Second Birthday is canon now. We plan to make a weekend
out of it. Starting with a proper celebration of Krystin's actual and only
birthday tonight. A do-over of the one we planned last year, same restaurant. Followed by an Easter egg hunt tomorrow morning and a trip to the
Mall of America for bubble tea with tapioca pearls. My idea.

I'm not rushing to get out of bed. I'm soaking in the giddy-nervous
feeling I have, like a universe is being born in my chest. I think I will
cry today.

Anna declares we shouldn't waste the day in bed and throws the comforter to our feet. I wiggle and whine but deep down agree. It becomes
too cold to just lie there so I get up and plug in my phone next to the
coffee maker, starting a pot while staring at the blank screen, waiting for
it to respawn after the battery died.

Multiple texts come in hard and fast.

Glad you're here, with a blue heart emoji from a number I don't
instantly recognize. It ends up being my sister Alyssa.

*I am so sorry, Paul. You are my son, and I would have done anything to
stop what happened.* Safe to assume this is Mom. She sends a follow-up.

Worst day of my life but best day of my life honey I'm so glad you're here and I'm so glad you're OK. I will never forget and have not forgotten. It is on my mind as much as you. Not a day goes by I don't thank God you're here, she types.

I so badly want to be cool today.

I throw on dressy clothes right before we leave. Black polo, black pants, and the same sharp gray suit jacket that I wore to my job interview and nailed it.

In the mirror, my hair is long again. Longer even than the day I got shot. I'm growing it out, hoping it will protect me in the future somehow. The incision scar makes an X with my natural part. Visibly breeching. I run my finger along the length of the scar. Starting just above my left ear, ending a little past the midway point on my head. As if I'm making it, right now, live and in person. As if I'm drawing a line in some dirt. *It is in the past*, I think, *and it is here too*. Coloring my present, morphing my future. All while I give it meaning. How weird. I put on my Superman socks and start to cry again.

At the restaurant, I keep an eye on the time. Our food comes out at 6:45. I sense a conversation about Krystin's new haircut and color is wrapping up. Then, I announce what was happening three hundred and sixty-five days ago this very instant.

"Three hundred and sixty-five days ago this very instant, I just got shot," I announce, feeling the back of my head, the phantom lump behind my ear, where I struck the chair. It is still sensitive to the touch a year later. Nerves don't forget either.

Everyone fidgets and thumbs their silverware. Mom texts me from across the table, *I feel bad about what you are saying right now*. She is sort of crying. I text back, *I know, but we should acknowledge it for a final scrap of closure*.

I need to turn the Ghost of April 7 into a Spirit. And it starts with this ceremony, reliving what happened to the minute, as a family, one last time. It needs to feel like a past life that I vaguely remember. A literal book on a shelf, read through once upon a time, with proper distance and due respect, that now is scarcely revisited.

"And look where we are now, bitches," my brother-in-law says.

Together. Because it is never guaranteed. Cliches go out the window once you've buddied up with death. Everyone toasts and cheers their glasses.

Krystin opens presents. I hand her a bag with some Tupperware covered by two sheets of Kleenex. In the Tupperware is a scrap of paper. Written on the scrap of paper is the following: *I know what this looks like. It looks like sloppy handwriting on a scrap of paper in some Tupperware. It looks like a last-minute gift. Though that may be true, it is also the gift of what you didn't get today, tomorrow. Anna and I will buy you any number of items at the Mall of America equal or up to the total value of $50. Happy Birthday!*

"Three hundred and sixty-five days ago this very instant," I say, "Mark was putting guns in his car and lying to a Public Safety officer." I could have been bleeding out in my bed, and he wouldn't have known the difference.

Mom reveals she has one more gift. She hands me a bag.

"For Easter. And your second birthday," she says. I smile at her use of the term. In the bag is a shirt with the logo of the *Daily Planet* across the front, the newspaper in the Superman universe. "It works for two reasons," Mom says. "You're Superman, and a writer." Underneath the shirt is a pile of KitKats, my favorite chocolate.

We sing "Happy Birthday" to Krystin while our waiter brings out a free ice cream sundae. Mom also brought raspberry cake that she made. I pick a full berry off the top.

"Three hundred and sixty-five days ago this very instant, I was bumming around a kitchen island with Mark and Keith, discussing how we should patch all the holes. The cops still haven't been called," I say.

Mom walks one of my nieces, now one year old, around the bar to work off some of the sugar. My other niece, now four and a half, comes by me and does magic tricks with a quarter that her dad gave her.

She tells me to close my eyes. I can tell she is shuffling for a place to hide the quarter. She rests it in a fold on my jacket and tells me to open my eyes.

I look for the quarter everywhere it's not.

"It must have disappeared," I say, playing the game. "I simply can't find it anywhere."

She plucks it out of the jacket fold. I'm shocked and dismayed, she is monster-phlegm laughing. She tells me to close my eyes again, and she hides the quarter in her fist, then a different fold on my jacket.

"Remind me to tell you why we are celebrating this weekend, like, fifteen years from now," I say as she walks back to her seat.

On the way home I remind Anna that the paramedics finally arrived.

During a *Ghost Adventures* marathon, I state that I just made it to the hospital.

While heating up a cup of decaffeinated green tea in the microwave, I get the results from my CT scan, I shout from the kitchen.

I say out loud to myself during my nightly sit-up routine that Mom, just now, knows I'm not dead, nor the mental equivalent. I text her that.

Showering, I tell my shampoo bottle that the rest of my family just showed up to the hospital. They love me very much, I tell the shampoo. I don't admit that enough. They love me, and I love them.

In bed, I poke Anna, who is already fast asleep, and whisper to the back of her head that three hundred and sixty-five days ago this very instant, I'm getting a tetanus shot in my butt.

Morning comes and I search for Easter eggs instead of the courage to accept surgery. I feel around for bright plastic shells instead of the hole in my head. People are touching my shoulder, mouthing, *Did you see the one in the lampshade?* Instead of, *See you when it's over. You'll be fine. I love you.*

I guess there are four hundred and one jelly beans in a jar instead of how long the operation will take and if I'll make it or not. My prize is a scratch-off lottery ticket, but I don't win any money.

"Three hundred and sixty-five days ago this very instant, I just woke up, and you all just ordered pizza," I say.

The shooting caused countless negative impacts that still ripple in its wake, largely related to my mental health, with a few cognitive and a few physical residual symptoms. But it has given me reasons to be better. I am more forgiving. I am more empathetic. I think more critically about basic human rights, basic human kindness. I have learned universal truths amid extreme circumstances. I have learned to value freedom, after I had none, trapped in my spiral-inducing trauma bubble for the better part of four years. I have learned to treasure my family, those who would do anything for me, and the time we spend together.

I am open, and not just because I have a new hole in my head. I am really open. Reading and writing are a far less violent way to achieve something similar. You, reader, have aided in my healing. You are an active participant. I hope along the way I've changed you, too, somehow. If that is the case, the outcome has finally transcended the incident itself. I can officially call myself a survivor and believe it.

I realize that nothing about my life has been wasted. Dramatically changed, yes, but I am grateful for a unique life, with its own brand of misfortune and opportunity. If we are hardheaded, strong-willed, we can adapt. If we can adapt, then we can fly. Maybe not like Superman, but in our own ways.

Metaphorically, everyone gets shot in the head. Sometimes it's a spit-ball, or a plastic BB. Sometimes it's a hollow-point 9mm. As a member of the human race, our future contains grievous damage, unbearable hurt, immeasurable trauma, sometimes from the people we least expect. But as I said to my mom the day of my second birthday, it was my challenge, my duty to heal. To try. To try my hardest. To allow myself to be hurt and ugly and hopeless—knowing that whatever happened, knowing that maybe the bullet could still win—I would trudge onward also knowing that someone or something was going to love me anyway. I looked at my mom and her eyes said, *That is so true.*

ACKNOWLEDGMENTS

Massive thanks to the literary magazines and editors who published pieces of this book in somewhat altered forms: Mensah Demary at *Catapult*, Scott Garson at *Wigleaf*, Megan Pillow at *The Audacity*, Donna Talarico and Steph Auteri at *Hippocampus Magazine*, Hannah Grieco at *JMWW*, Katherine Gehan at *Pithead Chapel*, Michael Wheaton at *Autofocus Literary*, Matthew Fleischer at the *San Francisco Chronicle*, and finally Crow Jonah and Aaron Burch at *HAD*. Thank you for championing my work and the work of our amazing literary community. This book wouldn't be the same without you.

A special thanks to Roxane Gay for publishing my piece "Public Safety" as the first essay in *The Audacity's* Emerging Writers Series. No one lifts up other writers quite like Roxane Gay. As a longtime student and fan of your work, the honor is tremendous.

Eternal gratitude to my agent, Michele Mortimer, who has been the best mentor, collaborator, resource, and advocate I could ever hope for. You believed in my story from the beginning, and after three years and about a thousand drafts, that belief never faltered. This book would not exist without your exceptional attention and care. I cannot wait to see what our creative partnership conjures up next.

I owe so much to my editor, Austin Ross, who took a chance on this book and shared my vision for it immediately. Your edits were so on-point—elevating and insightful—it made my words feel like a three-dimensional object to me for the first time. I'd also like to thank Josh, Hannah, Lauren, Kevin, Jenn and the entire team at Harper Horizon for their kindness, enthusiasm, and creativity in bringing this book to life.

To all the teachers, readers, friends, and strangers who have each contributed to this book in their own unique way: Salvatore Pane, Chris Santiago, George Saunders, Amber Sparks, James Tate Hill, Leslie Miller, Amy Muse, Hannah Brattesani, Jon, Leti, Nora, John, Al, Nick, JoAnn, Rick, Mary, Paul, Russel, Adriel, Eny, Matthew, Alex, Abby, Tara, CD Projekt Red, Greg Koch, Vintage Guitar Magazine, Blaire, Will, Austin, Hasan, Dane, Britt, Kyle, Chris, Jace, Jim Petersen, Michael Grady, and every Minnesota Timberwolves player ever, thank you, for real.

And lastly, to my entire family: Mom, Dad, Anna, Krystin, Alyssa, Lonny, Dan, Gary, Steve, Megan, Grandma Mary, my cats Mira and Mushroom (Mushy), and everyone else. It's only with your infinite love and support I was able to make this happen. This one goes out to you.

NOTES

CHAPTER 2

1. "Brain Injury Facts," International Brain Injury Association, Internationalbrain.org, accessed January 30, 2024, https://www.internationalbrain.org/resources/brain-injury-facts.
2. "Traumatic Brain Injury and Concussion: Get the Facts," Centers for Disease Control and Prevention, last reviewed April 20, 2023, https://www.cdc.gov/traumaticbraininjury/get_the_facts.html.
3. "Traumatic Brain Injury in the Workplace," Centers for Disease Control and Prevention, last reviewed October 16, 2023, https://www.cdc.gov/traumaticbraininjury/military/index.html.

CHAPTER 12

1. *Oxford English Dictionary*, s.v. "*grazed (v.),*" accessed April 16, 2024, https://www.oed.com/search/dictionary/?scope=Entries&q=grazed.

CHAPTER 41

1. Christopher Ingraham, "There are more guns than people in the United States, according to a new study of global firearm ownership," *Washington Post*, June 19, 2018, https://www.washingtonpost.com/news/wonk/wp/2018/06/19/there-are-more-guns-than-people-in-the-united-states-according-to-a-new-study-of-global-firearm-ownership/.

CHAPTER 78

1. J. Craig Oxman, "Clapton's Fool: History's Greatest Guitar?" *Vintage Guitar Magazine*, December 2011, https://www.vintageguitar.com/12684/claptons-fool/.

ABOUT THE AUTHOR

Paul Rousseau is a disabled writer with work in Roxane Gay's *The Audacity, Catapult, The San Francisco Chronicle*, and elsewhere. You can find more of his work online at Paul-Rousseau.com.